FIVE

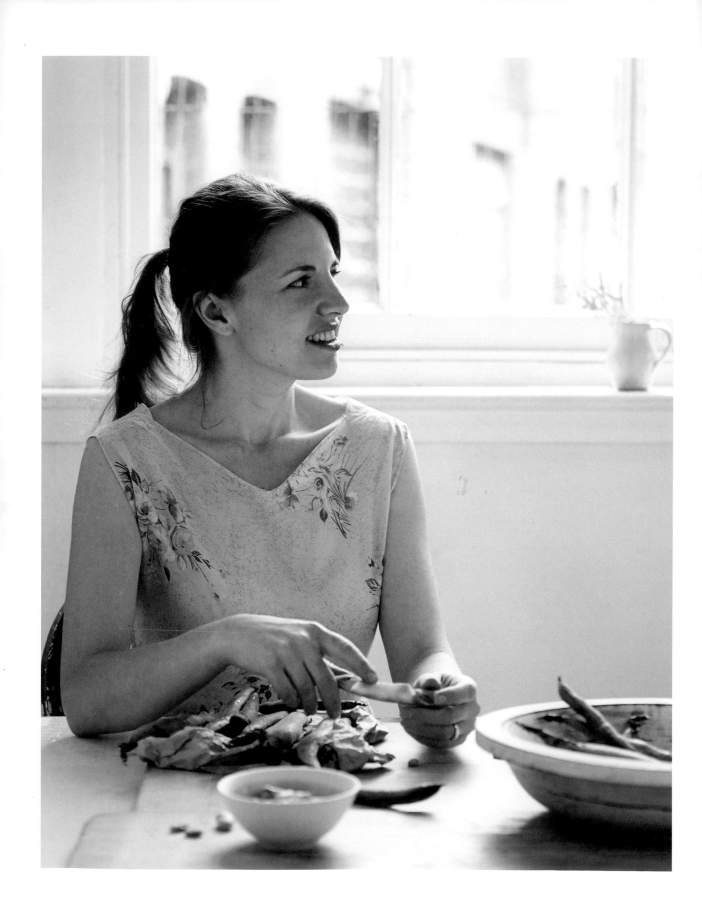

FIVE

RACHEL DE THAMPLE

EBURY
PRESS

10 9 8 7 6 5 4 3 2 1

Ebury Press, an imprint of Ebury Publishing,
20 Vauxhall Bridge Road,
London, SW1V 2SA

Ebury Press is part of the Penguin Random House group of companies whose
addresses can be found at global.penguinrandomhouse.com

Penguin
Random House
UK

Text © Rachel de Thample 2015
Photography by Nassima Rothacker © Ebury Press 2015

Rachel de Thample has asserted her right to be identified as the author of this Work
in accordance with the Copyright, Designs and Patents Act 1988.

First published by Ebury Press in 2015.

www.eburypublishing.co.uk
A CIP catalogue record for this book is available from the British Library

Editor: Rachel Malig
Design: Two Associates
Photography: Nassima Rothacker
Styling: Rachel de Thample and Nassima Rothacker

ISBN: 9780091959661

Colour reproduction by Altaimage
Printed and bound in China by Toppan Leefung

Penguin Random House is committed to a sustainable future for
our business, our readers and our planet. This book is made from
Forest Stewardship Council® certified paper

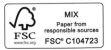

MIX
Paper from
responsible sources
FSC® C104723

CONTENTS

INTRODUCTION

Five is the bare minimum when it comes to how much fruit and veg we need to eat each day, but most of us are barely even eating half of this. We all know that eating more of the stuff keeps us healthy and alive, helps battles colds, ward off flu, increases cancer protection and makes us feel and look vibrant. So why aren't we eating more of the stuff? One of the key culprits is convenience.

I can't tell you how many times I've been walking around London on empty, craving what I know is healthy and good. The options are exactly opposite to what we need: sugary muffins, milky coffees, buttery croissants, pre-packed sandwiches, chocolate bars and fizzy drinks. How often do you see mounds of fresh fruit or punnets of veg? Perhaps I'm the only person in the world who'd do cartwheels along a train platform that had a fruit and veg vending machine. One day… In the meantime, you'll find me waiting for my train in Balham with a punnet of cherry tomatoes or tucking into a bag of peas – the perfect healthy portable snack. Just throw some into your bag before you leave the house. You can easily get two portions of veg simply by snacking. Rather than having a post carb crash, you'll have a sustained surge of energy.

When you're not out and about, I hope this book will provide you with heaps of inspiration to eat more fruit and veg than you ever have before. I have started with breakfast and taken you right through to dessert, with really simple but delicious recipes. Nearly every single recipe offers at least 1 portion of fruit and veg. Some dishes even give you five portions in a single serving.

While not a vegetarian book, the slant of the recipes is most certainly 'less meat, more veg', and there are many vegan options. I've also tried to cater to dietary requirements. Half way through writing the book, I had to start a rigid detox programme because I'd picked up a pesky parasite. I sought help from a nutritionist and she gave me a list of foods I needed to cut out (wheat, dairy and sugar). She also gave me a list of food TO EAT. A mountain of fruit and veg was at the top of her prescription, and it worked. Many of the dishes in the book were born out of my detox – not all, mind. I'm a firm believer in a healthy balance. We all need a slice of cake sometimes.

MENU IDEAS

Using this book can easily help you eat far more than five portions of fruit and veg a day. Here are just a few delicious examples.

Breakfast

Fig, Almond and Orange Blossom Muffins
    (1 portion)

Clementine and Saffron Tea (1 portion)

Lunch

Coconut Crab Coronation Slaw (2 portions)

Weekend dinner

Cauliflower Couscous with Coriander and
    Orange (2.5 portions)

Warming Tunisian Stew with Smoked Fish
    (3 portions)

Plum and Liquorice Jelly (1 portion)

= 10.5 portions in a day

Breakfast

Summer Berry Crush (2 portions)

Fig, Rose and Coconut Breakfast Truffles
    (1 portion)

Lunch

Moroccan Beetroot Soup with Mint Labneh
    (3.5 portions)

Sassy Cherry and Watercress Salad with
    Crushed Pistachios (2 portions)

Dinner

Summer Tomato and Bean Curry with
    Cumin Dosas (4 portions)

Saffron Ice Crème with Strawberries
    (1 portions)

−13.5 portions in a day

Breakfast

Apple Strudel Galette (2 portions)

Lunch

Sticky Ginger Pumpkin with Butter Bean
    Dal (5 portions)

Dinner

The Zingy Tahini Dress with a selection
    of dipping veg (1 portion)

Chard Dolmades with Little Fish
    (2 portions)

Mulled Figs with Mascarpone (1 portion)

− 11 portions in a day

Breakfast

A Coffee Date (1.5 portions)

Lunch

Honeyed Parsnip Quinoa with Chilli,
    Cardamom and Orange (4 portions)

Dinner

Winter Roots and Leaves Salad with
    Tropical Dressing (2 portions)

Ali's Caribbean Curry with Coconut
    Crusted Fish (2 portions)

Rebel's Hop Banoffee (1 portion)

= 10.5 portions in a day

FIVE FRUIT AND VEGETABLES

WHAT EQUALS A PORTION?

Apple	1 medium apple
Apricot	2 fresh or 2 dried apricots
Asparagus	5 chunky or 8–10 thin spears
Aubergine	⅓ aubergine
Avocado	1 small or ½ large avocado
Bananas	1 small banana
Beansprouts	4 tbsp sprouts
Beetroot	½ large or 1 small beetroot
Black beans	5 tbsp cooked black beans
Blackberries	7 large or 9 small berries
Blueberries	½ cup or 30 berries
Broad beans	5 tbsp or beans from 7–8 pods
Broccoli	5 chunky florets
Brussels sprouts	5 sprouts
Butter beans	5 tbsp cooked butter beans
Butternut squash	¼ medium squash
Cabbage	⅛ head of cabbage
Carrot	1 medium or 2 small carrots
Cauliflower	5 florets
Celeriac	⅛ celeriac
Celery	2 sticks of celery
Chard	2 leaves of chard
Cherries	10 cherries
Chickpeas	5 tbsp cooked chickpeas
Chicory	½ head of chicory
Chinese leaf	3 leaves
Clementine	2 clementines
Cranberries	about 20 fresh berries, or 1 tbsp dried cranberries
Courgette	½ courgette
Cucumber	⅓ large or ½ smaller cucumber
Currants (red, black and white)	5 tbsp fresh currants
Dandelion greens	2 large handfuls of greens
Dates	2 dates
Fennel	⅓ fennel
Figs	1 plump fresh fig or 2 dried figs
Flat beans	a fist full of beans for 7 beans
French beans	a fist full of beans or 14 beans
Globe artichokes	1 freshly cooked globe arichoke or 2 marinated artichoke hearts
Gooseberries	½ cup or 15 gooseberries
Grapefruit	½ large grapefruit
Grapes	15 grapes
Jerusalem artichokes	4 large Jerusalem artichokes
Kale	3 tbsp finely chopped kale or 2 whole leaves
Kiwi fruit	2 kiwis
Kohlrabi	½ kohlrabi
Leek	½ leek
Lemon	150ml juice
Lentils	5 tbsp cooked lentils
Lettuce	4–5 large lettuce leaves or 1 cup smaller leaves
Mangetout	10 mangetout
Mango	⅓ mango
Marrow	⅛ marrow
Melon	⅓ melon

Mushrooms	1 portobello mushroom, 6 chestnut or button mushrooms, or 1 large handful wild mushrooms
Nasturtium leaves and flowers	2 large handfuls of leaves and/or flowers
Nectarine	1 large or 2 small nectarines
Okra	8 whole okra
Onions	1 medium onion
Orange	1 orange
Pak choi	3 larger or 4 smaller pak choi leaves
Parsnips	1 medium-sized parsnip
Peaches	1 peach
Pears	1 small pear
Peas	5 tbsp fresh or frozen peas
Peppers	½ large pepper or 1 small pepper
Pineapple	A 3cm-thick slice of pineapple
Plums	2 plums
Pomegranate	½ pomegranate
Porcini	2 large fresh porcini (ceps) or a small handful of dried
Prunes	2 prunes
Pumpkin	⅙ large, ¼ medium or 1 mini pumpkin
Quince	½ quince
Radicchio	3 radicchio leaves
Radish	5 radishes
Raisins	1 heaped tbsp raisins
Raspberries	5 tbsp or about 20 berries
Red cabbage	⅛ head of cabbage
Rhubarb	2 sticks of rhubarb
Rocket	2 large handfuls of rocket
Runner beans	3 runner beans
Salsify	2 sticks of salsify
Samphire	½ cup samphire
Shallots	4 small shallots or 1 banana shallot
Sorrel	1 cup sorrel
Spinach	3 large handfuls raw spinach or ½ cup cooked spinach
Spring greens	3 larger spring green leaves or ½ cup chopped spring greens
Spring onions	3 spring onions
Squash	½ smaller summer squash or ⅙ medium-sized autumnal (pumpkin-like squash)
Strawberries	5 berries
Sugar snap peas	15 peas
Swede	⅙ larger or ¼ smaller swede
Sweet potato	½ sweet potato
Sweetcorn	1 full cob of sweetcorn or ½ cup kernals
Tomato	1 medium tomato or 7 cherry tomatoes
Watercress	1 cup watercress
Watermelon	⅙ small watermelon

BREAKFAST

Muffins

THE BASICS: Fruit and veg hugely improve the texture of muffins and cakes, not only adding moistness, but also sweetness and extra flavour. The key is getting the balance right. You don't want the batter too runny or too stiff, but somewhere right in the middle. Don't overmix your batter. The wet and dry ingredients must be mixed separately first and then gently folded together – never whisked or stirred. Lastly, make sure your baking powder and bicarbonate of soda are within their use-by date; your bakes will flop if they've expired. Another tip is tapping. Once you've filled your muffin or cake tin, give it a few taps on a work surface. Not only does this even the tops, but it prevents the raising agents from acting before they need to.

Always leave muffins to cool for 10–15 minutes before eating – this allows all the steam to escape, giving the muffins a better texture.

APPLE PEANUT BUTTER

 JUST UNDER 1 PORTION
PER MUFFIN

PREP	15 MINS
COOK	20 MINS
MAKES	8 MEDIUM-SIZED MUFFINS

4 tbsp peanut butter, chunky or smooth (or swap for your favourite nut butter – almond's a good choice)

6 tbsp sugar (caster, brown, demerara, coconut palm)

1 egg, beaten

1 tsp vanilla extract

150ml apple juice

400g apples, coarsely grated (I don't bother peeling them)

1 tsp baking powder

½ tsp bicarbonate of soda

200g wholegrain flour (wheat, spelt, kamut, rye)

8–12 thin apple slices, cored (i.e. raw apple rings)

Preheat the oven to 180°C/Gas 4. Lightly oil a muffin tin or use paper liners.

In a large bowl, beat the peanut butter and sugar until nicely mixed. Whisk in the egg, vanilla and apple juice, then add the apples, baking powder and bicarbonate of soda and mix well.

Tip the flour in. Gently fold the flour through the wet ingredients with a large spoon or spatula until just incorporated.

Spoon the mixture into the prepared muffin tin, dividing it equally among eight holes or paper liners. As a finishing touch, crown each muffin with an apple ring, gently pressing it into the batter so it nestles on top.

Tap the muffin tin firmly on the work surface three times before placing in the oven (middle shelf, set in the centre). Bake for about 20 minutes, or until golden on top and cooked through. Pierce with a small knife or toothpick through the centre to test; it should come out clean.

PEAR, HAZELNUT AND HONEYED GOAT'S CURD

 JUST UNDER 1 PORTION PER MUFFIN

PREP   15 MINS
COOK   20 MINS
MAKES 8 MEDIUM-SIZED MUFFINS

4 tbsp olive or hazelnut oil

6 tbsp sugar (caster, brown, demerara, coconut palm)

1 egg, beaten

½ tsp ground cinnamon (plus extra for the tops)

150ml apple or pear juice

1 sprig of fresh rosemary, leaves finely chopped (optional)

1 tsp baking powder

½ tsp bicarbonate of soda

400g pears, coarsely grated (I don't bother peeling them)

100g hazelnuts, crushed and toasted

200g wholegrain flour (wheat, spelt, rye, kamut)

FOR THE TOPPING
2 tsp runny honey

a pinch of ground cinnamon

100g goat's curd (or any similar mild, soft, creamy cheese)

100g natural or Greek yoghurt

Preheat the oven to 180°C/Gas 4. Lightly oil a muffin tin or use paper liners.

Beat the oil, sugar and egg together until smooth and creamy. Whisk in the cinnamon and juice. Add the rosemary, (if using, baking powder and bicarbonate of soda and mix to combine, then fold in the grated pears and half the hazelnuts.

Tip in the flour. Gently fold the flour through the wet ingredients with a large spoon or spatula until just incorporated. Spoon the mix into the prepared muffin tin, dividing it equally among eight holes or paper liners.

Tap the muffin tin firmly on the work surface three times before placing in the oven (middle shelf, set in the centre). Bake for about 20 minutes, or until golden on top and cooked through. Pierce with a small knife or toothpick through the centre to test; it should come out clean.

For the goat's curd topping, fold the honey, cinnamon, curd (or similar cheese) and yoghurt together. Top the muffins with the sweetened cheese and finish with the remaining toasted hazelnuts and a dusting of cinnamon.

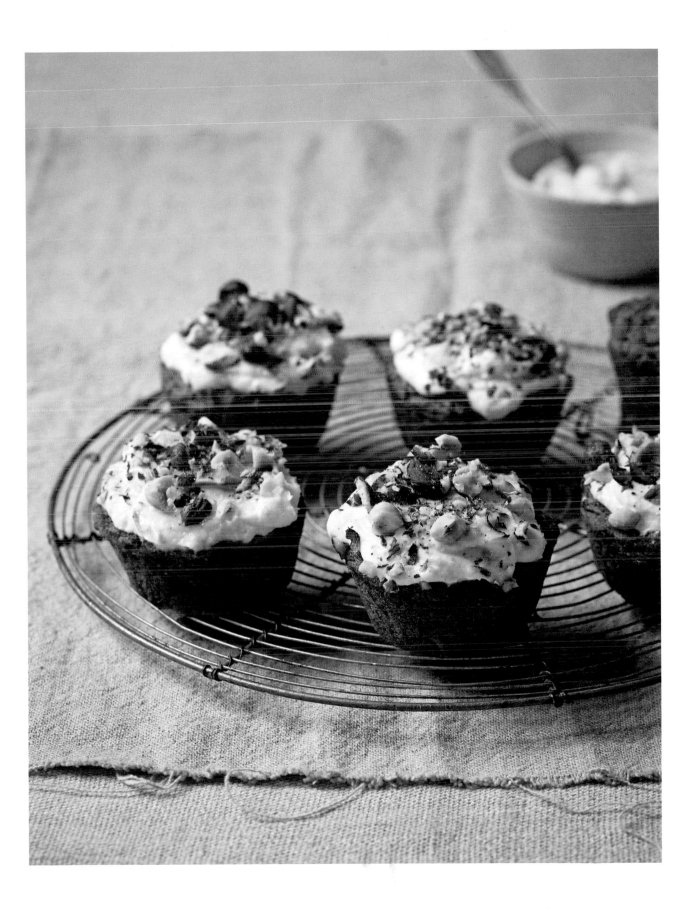

FIG, ALMOND AND ORANGE BLOSSOM

The orange blossom water really adds something special to these muffins but, that said, if you can't find or don't have any, they most certainly can be made without.

 JUST UNDER 1 PORTION PER MUFFIN

PREP   10 MINS
COOK   20 MINS
MAKES 8 MEDIUM-SIZED MUFFINS

12 dried figs

4 tbsp olive oil

6 tbsp runny honey

1 egg, beaten

1 tsp vanilla extract

1 tbsp orange blossom water

1 tsp ground cinnamon

10 cardamom pods, seeds finely ground

2 oranges

1 tsp baking powder

½ tsp bicarbonate of soda

150g ground almonds

50g wholegrain (wheat, spelt, rye, kamut) or gluten-free flour

a handful of whole almonds, to garnish

Trim the tough tip from the fig stems. Place the figs in a saucepan with enough water to cover. Boil for 5 minutes, or until the figs have plumped up. Drain the figs. Finely chop until you have a figgy paste. Preheat the oven to 180°C/Gas 4. Lightly oil a muffin tin or use paper liners.

Beat the oil and honey together in a bowl until nicely mixed. Whisk in the egg, vanilla, orange blossom water, cinnamon and ground cardamom.

Grate in the zest from the oranges. Squeeze out 150ml juice. Add the juice to the mix, along with the fig paste, baking powder and bicarbonate of soda. Whisk to combine. Add the ground almonds and flour to the wet ingredients. Gently fold through with a large spoon or spatula until just mixed.

Spoon the mix into the prepared muffin tin, dividing it equally among eight holes or paper liners. Tap the tin firmly on the countertop three times. Decorate the tops with whole almonds – I like to arrange them in a circle like flower petals.

Bake in the oven (middle shelf, set in the centre) for about 20 minutes, or until golden on top and cooked through. Pierce with a small knife or toothpick through the centre to test; it should come out clean.

Variation: turn your muffin mix into a tea-time loaf. Just pour into a medium-sized loaf tin or a few mini ones. Bake for about 45–60 minutes, or until golden on top and set in the middle.

BLACKCURRANT CRUMBLE

 JUST UNDER 1 PORTION PER MUFFIN

PREP   15 MINS
COOK   20 MINS
MAKES 8 MEDIUM-SIZED MUFFINS

FOR THE MUFFINS
4 tbsp oil (olive, rapeseed, coconut, almond)

6 tbsp sugar (caster, brown, demerara, coconut palm)

1 egg, beaten

1 tsp vanilla extract or seeds from ½ vanilla pod

150ml apple or orange juice

1 tsp baking powder

½ tsp bicarbonate of soda

300g black or redcurrants (pulled from their stems)

200g wholegrain flour (kamut flour is lovely in this one)

FOR THE TOPPING
3 tbsp wholegrain flour

2 tbsp sugar

a pinch of ground cinnamon

1 tbsp oil (the same used for the muffins)

Preheat the oven to 180°C/Gas 4. Lightly oil a muffin tin or use paper liners.

For the crumble topping, mix the flour, sugar and cinnamon together in a bowl. Drizzle the oil over and mix with your fingers until it resembles wet sand.

For the muffins, beat the oil and sugar together in a bowl until nicely mixed. Whisk in the egg, vanilla and fruit juice until well incorporated. Add the baking powder and bicarbonate of soda and mix to combine, then fold in the currants.

Tip the flour in. Gently fold the flour through the wet ingredients with a large spoon or spatula until just incorporated.

Spoon the mix into the prepared muffin tin, filling it until ¾ full. Dust each muffin with enough crumble topping to generously cover.

Tap the muffin tin firmly on the work surface three times before placing in the oven (middle shelf, set in the centre). Bake for about 20 minutes, or until golden on top and cooked through. Pierce with a small knife or toothpick through the centre to test; it should come out clean.

When warm, these muffins can be a little gooey due to all that lovely fruit packed inside. I prefer to let them cool fully before removing them from the tin.

BUZZY BANANA

 JUST UNDER 1 PORTION PER MUFFIN

PREP	15 MINS
COOK	20 MINS
MAKES	8 MEDIUM-SIZED MUFFINS

4 large or 6 smaller ripe bananas

4 tbsp oil (olive, coconut, walnut)

1 egg, beaten

6 tbsp sugar (caster, brown, demerara, coconut palm)

1 tsp vanilla extract

150ml freshly brewed coffee

1 tsp baking powder

½ tsp bicarbonate of soda

200g wholegrain flour (wheat, spelt, kamut, rye)

a large handful of walnuts, toasted (optional)

Preheat the oven to 180°C/Gas 4. Lightly oil a muffin tin or use paper liners.

Mash the bananas in a bowl until you have a fairly smooth purée. Whisk the oil and egg into the bananas, then beat in the sugar, vanilla and coffee.

Sprinkle the baking powder and bicarbonate of soda over the top and mix to combine. Tip in the flour and gently fold through using a large spoon or spatula until it is just incorporated. Fold in half of the walnuts, if using.

Spoon the mix into the prepared muffin tin, filling it until ¾ full. Dot the tops with the remaining walnuts.

Tap the muffin tin firmly on the work surface three times before placing in the oven (middle shelf, set in the centre). Bake for about 20 minutes, or until golden on top and cooked through. Pierce with a small knife or toothpick through the centre to test; it should come out clean.

Fruity Teas

THE BASICS: A little fresh juice or chopped fruit (fresh or dried) can easily be transformed into a gorgeous tea with a little spice and hot water, as the following ideas illustrate.

WILD ROSEHIP

Rosehips are the stunning red fruits found on rosebushes in the autumn, but they also linger right through the winter. I always wait until the first frost before I pick them, and I only go for ones that are squishy. You can just squeeze the orangey-red paste (used to make this tea) right out as if it were toothpaste. Rosehips are packed full of vitamin C and they have a magical taste, as if you're sipping a medieval brew.

PORTION PER POT

PREP   15 MINS
COOK   10–15 MINS
MAKES   1 LARGE POT

350g ripe, wild rosehips

a pot of boiling water

a little honey, to taste

Rinse your rosehips. Place in a saucepan. Pour in enough water to just barely cover. Simmer for 10 minutes. If the rosehips are hard, you'll need to simmer for a little longer, until they become mushably soft.

Smash the rosehips with a fork to extract their pulp and lovely colour. Strain through a muslin cloth, squeezing out as much pulp as you can.

Once you have a purée of rosehips, spoon the purée into a tea pot. Top up with a good splash of boiling water and a swirl of honey. Taste. Add more water or honey, until it's just right for you.

If you accidently dilute it too much, turn the muslin cloth with your rosehip pulp into a tea bag. Just tie it up to secure it and pop it into the pot to infuse.

SPICED APRICOT

PORTION PER POT

PREP   5 MINS
COOK   10 MINS
MAKES   ENOUGH FOR 4–6

12 dried apricots

a pot of boiling water

a hint of spice• (optional)

Place the apricots in a small saucepan with just enough boiling water to cover. Simmer for 10 minutes, or until the apricots are plump and tender enough to purée.

Whizz the apricots with the cooking water until you have a smooth paste. Trickle in more water little by little, until the tea is as thick or thin, strong or weak as you like it. I like it about as thick as Turkish coffee. Add a hint of spice, if desired, and serve.

• *Warming spices like cloves, ginger, nutmeg, cinnamon and/or allspice all work beautifully.*

CLEMENTINE AND SAFFRON

 PORTION PER POT

PREP 5 MINS
COOK 5 MINS
MAKES 1 SMALL POT

2 whole clementines

a pinch of saffron threads

300ml boiling water

a little honey, to taste
(optional)

Halve the clementines, then squeeze the juice into a tea pot. Pop the squeezed clementine halves into the pot as well with a pinch of saffron threads.

Pour in the hot water and let it steep for 5 minutes. Swirl in a little honey, to taste, and serve.

NOTE: You can also make this tea with normal oranges, but they're usually not quite as sweet so you may need that drop of honey.

APPLE, CARDAMOM AND FENNEL

 PORTION PER POT

PREP 5 MINS
COOK 5 MINS
MAKES 1 SMALL POT

150ml apple juice

150ml water

4 cardamom pods, crushed

a pinch of fennel seeds

stalks and ferny fronds from
1 fennel bulb (optional)

Pour the juice and water into a saucepan. Add the crushed cardamom pods and fennel seeds and bring to a gentle rolling boil.

Tuck the fennel stalks and fronds into a tea pot, if using. Pour the warm spiced apple mix into the pot and let it steep for a few minutes before serving. Deliciously soothing.

GRAPEFRUIT AND GINGER

 PORTION PER POT

PREP 5 MINS
COOK 5 MINS
MAKES 1 SMALL POT

1 grapefruit

5 thin slices of fresh ginger

300ml boiling water

a little honey, to taste
(optional)

Halve the grapefruit, then squeeze the juice into a tea pot. Pop the squeezed halves into the pot.

Bruise the ginger a little for a feistier ginger kick; just bash it in a pestle and mortar or place on a cutting board and crush the slices with the bottom of a jam jar. Add the ginger to the tea pot.

Pour in the hot water and let it steep for 5 minutes. Swirl in a little honey, to taste, and serve.

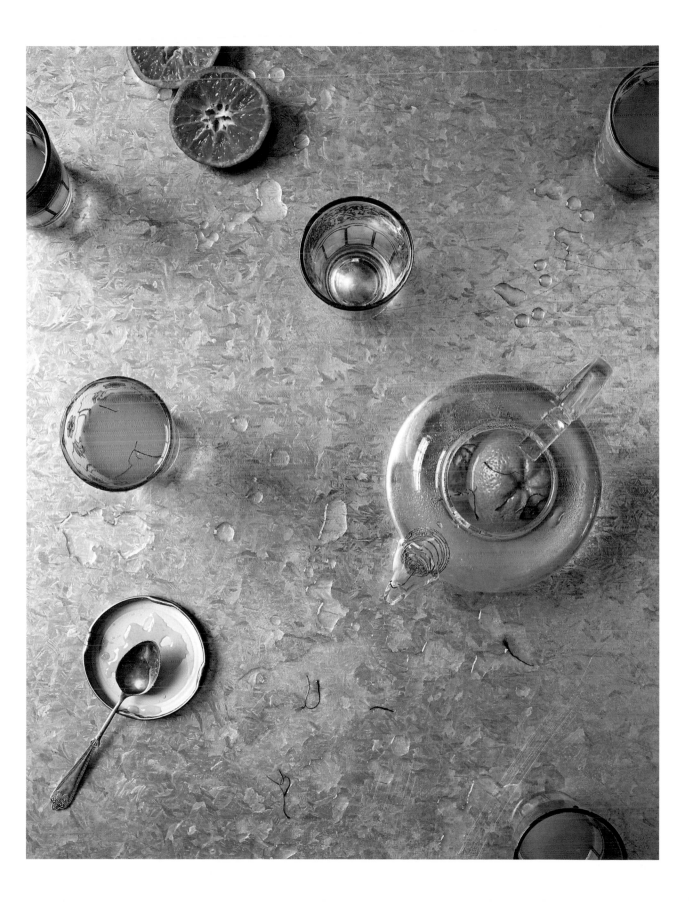

Galettes

THE BASICS: Around the corner from my old flat there was a cosy creperie, La Galette, where they served the most delicious Breton-style buckwheat pancakes. All washed down with Breton cider, of course.

Galettes are great carriers for all manner of filling, including lots of fruit and veg. Making your batter the night before and prepping your fillings means you can get breakfast on the table with little fuss. Allowing the batter to mature overnight also results in a lighter, more workable mix. If you want an instant buckwheat pancake fix, try the blinis on page 52.

GALETTE BATTER

PREP   **15 MINS (PLUS OVERNIGHT RESTING)**
COOK   **25 MINS**
MAKES   **4–6 GALETTES**

200g buckwheat flour

a pinch of sea salt

200ml hot water

2 tbsp butter or olive oil

200ml milk (any kind)

1 egg, beaten

50ml beer • (or water)

a few glosses of oil

Measure the flour into a large bowl and swirl in a good pinch of sea salt.

Mix the hot water and butter or oil until the butter melts. Pour into the flour along with the milk and egg and whisk until smooth. Pop the batter into the fridge and leave it to rest overnight. If you store it in a large jar or yoghurt pot with a lid, when you take it out of the fridge the next morning you can just give it a shake and pour it straight into the pan.

When you are ready to cook, add the beer or water to the batter and shake or whisk vigorously to mix.

Heat a large frying pan and brush with a little oil, just enough to coat. Pour the batter into the centre of the pan until you have a circle about the size of a saucer. Swirl the pan to distribute the batter thinly around the base (now it should be about the size of a dinner plate). Add a little more batter if needed but work quickly.

Cook over a high heat until golden. Flip, then spoon your filling into the centre. Once the underside is cooked, fold in the sides, leaving a little opening for the filling to peep out.

Use a sturdy spatula or two to transfer to a plate. Serve immediately, or pop in the oven on a low heat (100°C/Gas ½) to keep warm while you cook the others.

NOTE: The batter freezes well, or you can keep it in the fridge for a couple of days. Just make sure you shake or whisk well before using.

> ● *I like to use a red ale, one that has sweet, toasty, malty caramel notes, which enriches the flavours of the buckwheat. Whisking in water instead works just fine.*

The Fillings

CARAMELISED ONION FONDUE

 PORTION PER GALETTE

PREP 15 MINS
COOK 30 MINS
SERVES 4

a few glosses of olive oil

4 onions, thinly sliced

200g raclette, Comté or Gruyère cheese (Caerphilly also works a treat), grated

½ garlic clove, grated or finely chopped

1 tsp cornflour or plain white flour

150ml cider or a slightly sweet white wine like Riesling

4 sprigs of fresh thyme, plus extra to serve

1 x quantity of galette batter (see opposite)

sea salt and freshly ground black pepper

Heat a large frying pan and add a gloss of olive oil. Tumble in the sliced onions with a pinch of salt and pepper. Cook over a medium-low heat until meltingly tender, golden and sweet, about 15 minutes. While they cook, toss the grated cheese with the garlic and flour.

Warm the cider or wine in a saucepan until bubbling. Turn the heat to low then slowly add the cheese, stirring in a zigzag pattern as you add it to prevent it from clumping. Once the cheese is fully melted, take the pan off the heat. Add a little pepper, to taste.

Scatter the leaves from a sprig or two of thyme over the onions and mix through. Cook for a further minute, then remove from the heat.

Heat a separate frying pan and brush with a little oil, to coat. Prepare and cook a galette as described (see opposite). Once it is set on one side, flip, then tumble a quarter of the onions into the centre. Drizzle a quarter of the cheese over the top. Fold the sides of the galette in like a parcel and carefully transfer to a plate. Repeat with the remaining batter and filling.

Finish each galette with a scattering of thyme leaves and black pepper, if desired.

Variation: salute the changing seasons by finishing this galette with griddled asparagus when its time arrives, or you can tuck hunks of roasted squash into the galette along with the onions and cheese, adding a further portion of veg per serving.

TURKISH SPINACH

 1.5 PORTIONS
PER GALETTE

PREP	15 MINS
COOK	15 MINS
SERVES	4

500g spinach

2 garlic cloves, finely chopped

1 x quantity of galette batter (see page 20)

a few glosses of oil

100g natural or Greek yoghurt

2 tsp harissa or 1–2 tsp chilli flakes (more or less, to taste)

4 egg yolks

2 tbsp dukka

sea salt and freshly ground pepper

Heat a large pan or pot until hot while you prepare the spinach.

Use baby or small leaves of spinach if you can. If you've huge green leaves, strip off the woody stems (retain and use them in something else) and roughly chop the soft greens. Rinse the spinach, leaving the water clinging to the leaves. Add them to the hot pan along with a hit of salt and pepper, and the garlic. Fold the spinach until about half of it has wilted down; the rest will continue cooking after you've taken it off the heat. Tip the spinach into a sieve or colander. Gently squeeze it to remove the bitter juices.

Heat a separate frying pan and brush with a little oil, to coat. Prepare and cook a galette as described on page 20. Once it is set on one side, flip, then pile a mound of spinach in the centre. Top with a couple of tablespoons of yoghurt, a swirl of harissa or a pinch of chilli flakes.

Perch an egg yolk in the centre and scatter a little of the dukka mix on top. Fold the sides of the galette in toward and slightly over the filling, leaving a little peeping gap for the egg yolk. Pop a lid over the folded galette to help set the yolk to your liking. Transfer to a plate and repeat with the remaining batter and filling.

> **HOMEMADE DUKKA**
> Make your own dukka by toasting the following in a dry frying pan until fragrant: 2 tbsp sesame seeds, 1 tbsp cumin seeds, 1 tbsp coriander seeds, 2 tbsp pine nuts or crushed hazelnuts, a good pinch of sea salt. Store in a jam jar, lid tightly sealed, for up to 6 months.

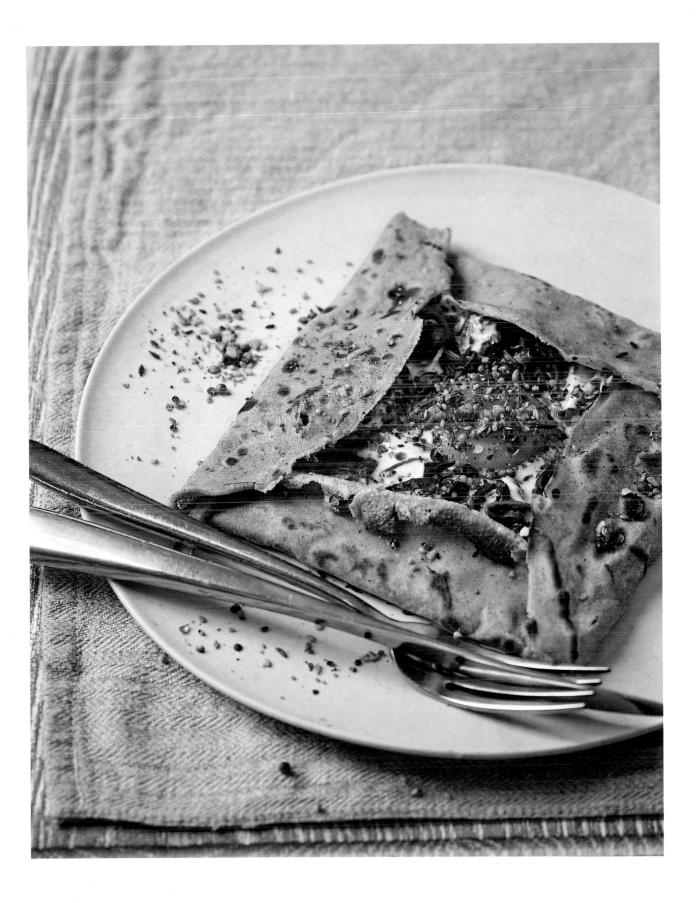

ENGLISH BREAKFAST

 PORTIONS PER GALETTE

PREP **20** MINS
COOK **40** MINS
SERVES **4**

a few glosses of olive or rapeseed oil

500g mushrooms, thinly sliced

4 rashers of smoked streaky bacon

8–12 cherry tomatoes, halved

2 garlic cloves, finely chopped

1 tsp marmite

a handful of fresh parsley, finely chopped

1 x quantity of galette batter (see page 20)

4 egg yolks

sea salt and freshly ground black pepper

Preheat the oven to 200°C/Gas 6. Place a large grill pan or roasting tin in the oven on the top shelf to heat up.

Warm a large frying pan and add a gloss of oil. Tumble in the mushrooms, then add a hit of pepper (skip the salt as the marmite will cover that). Sizzle until golden, about 10 minutes, adding more oil if needed.

While they cook, arrange your bacon and tomatoes, cut-side up, on your preheated grill pan or roasting tin. Place back on the top shelf. Roast for 15–20 minutes, or until the tomatoes are blistered and soft, and the bacon is crisp.

Once the mushrooms are golden, throw in the garlic. Cook for a moment, then fold in the marmite. Sizzle for a second until the marmite has coated the mushrooms in a sticky glaze. Toss in the parsley and set aside. Spoon the mushrooms into a dish. Give your pan a wash and put it back on the heat to make your galettes.

Brush the pan with a little oil, to coat. Prepare and cook a galette as described (see page 20). Once it is set on one side, flip, then scatter a quarter of the mushrooms in the centre.

Make a little indentation to hold an egg yolk and drop one in. I normally crack the eggs as each galette is ready, collecting the whites in a lidded container (to store in the fridge), and using my hands or the shell to cradle the yolk.

Fold the sides of your galette in like a parcel and let it cook for a moment to bring some of the heat to the yolk, just setting it. You can pop a lid over the galette to set it further, if desired.

Transfer to a plate and repeat with the remaining batter and filling.

To serve, sprinkle a little salt and pepper on the yolk. Drape the bacon over the edge of the galette and dot the tomatoes alongside.

NOTE: Serve the galettes with a glass of juice to bump the fruit up to 3 servings.

CINNAMON CHOCOLATE CHERRY

 PORTIONS PER GALETTE

PREP 15 MINS
COOK 30 MINS
SERVES 4

500g fresh cherries, stems and stones removed

250ml water

100g dark chocolate, chopped

a good pinch of ground cinnamon

35ml warm water (not boiling hot)

1 x quantity of galette batter (see page 20)

a few glosses of oil

a little mascarpone or goat's curd, to serve (optional)

Heat a saucepan or frying pan until hot. Add the cherries and water. Sizzle until the cherries have just started to soften and the water is almost gone; trickle in more water if it looks dry.

While the cherries cook, place the chocolate in a heatproof bowl. Stir the warm water into the chocolate, stirring until the chocolate is melted and glossy. If it's not fully melted, place the bowl over a saucepan of just-boiled water. Add the cinnamon, to taste.

Swirl the chocolate through the warm cherries once they're tender and have just a gloss of water remaining.

Heat a separate frying pan and brush with a little oil, to coat. Prepare and cook a galette as described on page 20. Once it is set on one side, flip, then mount a quarter of the chocolate cherries in the centre of the galette and fold the sides in like a parcel. Alternatively, fold it first and then pour the cherries and chocolate sauce over the top. Carefully transfer to a plate and repeat with the remaining batter and filling.

Top the galettes with a spoonful of mascarpone or goat's curd, if desired.

APPLE STRUDEL

 PORTIONS PER GALETTE

PREP 15 MINS
COOK 15 MINS
SERVES 4

8 apples, peeled, cored and finely diced

1 tsp vanilla extract

2 tsp ground cinnamon, plus extra for serving

1–2 tbsp maple syrup, plus extra for drizzling

1 x quantity of galette batter (see page 20)

natural or Greek yoghurt or mascarpone mixed with a scraping of vanilla seeds

a small handful of walnuts or flaked almonds, toasted

Tumble the apples and vanilla into a saucepan. Add a splash of water. Cook over a medium heat for 10–15 minutes, topping up with just enough water to prevent the apples from sticking to the pan. Once the apples are mashably soft, swirl in the cinnamon and 1 tablespoon of the maple syrup. Cook for a minute or two longer. Add a little more spice or sweetener, to taste.

Heat a separate frying pan and brush with a little oil, to coat. Prepare and cook a galette as described (see page 20). Once it is set on one side, flip, then dollop a quarter of the filling in the centre. Fold in the sides of the galette like a parcel and carefully transfer to a plate. Repeat with the remaining batter and filling.

Top each galette with a little vanilla yoghurt or mascarpone, a dusting of cinnamon, some toasted nuts and a good drizzle of syrup.

Veg Eggs

THE BASICS: There are no great formulas or philosophies here beyond the fact that eggs and veg are great bedfellows. I can think of few veg that you can't pair with eggs, whether in a frittata, omelette, hash, or veg on toast with a poached or fried egg on top. The following recipes will equip you with a few techniques and ideas to help you create your own variations using what's in season or in your fridge.

LEMONY SCRAMBLED EGGS WITH INDIAN SPICED SPINACH AND MUSHROOMS

2 PORTIONS PER SERVING

PREP 20 MINS
COOK 40 MINS
SERVES 4

8 eggs, beaten

1 lemon

a few glosses of olive oil

400g mushrooms, thinly sliced

3 garlic cloves, finely chopped

1 tbsp freshly grated ginger

a pinch of chilli powder (more or less, to taste)

1 tbsp cumin seeds, plus extra to garnish

1 tbsp powdered turmeric or 2 tbsp freshly grated

300g spinach, washed and roughly chopped if the leaves are large

sea salt and freshly ground black pepper

Place the eggs in a large bowl and grate in the zest of the lemon. Add a squeeze of lemon juice and a hit of salt and pepper. Whisk and set aside.

Heat a large frying pan and gloss with a little oil. Add the mushrooms, season with salt and pepper, and sizzle over a medium-high heat until the mushrooms are golden, about 10 minutes.

While the mushrooms are cooking, gloss the bottom of a small frying pan with just enough oil to coat. Add the eggs and cook over a low heat, folding the mix every time the eggs set on the bottom; I like mine a little on the runny side.

Swirl the garlic, ginger, chilli powder and spices into the mushrooms. Cook for a moment, then pile the spinach into the pan with a splash of water and fold through. Remove from the heat as soon as the spinach is tender, bright green and glossy. Finish with a squeeze of lemon juice and season to taste.

Pile the spiced veg on a plate and top with a mound of scrambled eggs. Scatter a pinch of cumin seeds over the top. Delicious served with warm naan or the Cumin Chana Dosas on page 129.

> ● *The spinach leaves can be swapped for chard, kale or cavolo nero. Remove large and woody stalks, chop the leaves roughly and cook as above. You can even use rocket or watercress, adding these to the mushrooms once you've taken them off the heat.*

TURKISH BAKED EGGS ON ROAST TOMATO TOASTS

 2 PORTIONS
PER SERVING

PREP   10 MINS
COOK   30–40 MINS
SERVES 4

4 thick slices of sourdough
   or ciabatta

a gloss of olive oil

500g cherry tomatoes,
   halved

4 eggs

100ml natural yoghurt

4 spring onions, chopped

a good pinch of chilli flakes
   (more or less, to taste)

sea salt and freshly ground
   black pepper

Preheat the oven to 180°C/Gas 4.

Arrange the slices of bread snugly in individual baking dishes (use a mini muffin loaf tin) or a small rectangular baking tray. Gloss the bread with a little oil.

Pile the halved tomatoes on top and season with a good pinch of salt and pepper.

Roast for 25–30 minutes, or until the tomatoes are tender and have deepened in colour. All their watery juices should have cooked down and concentrated. If not, cook a little longer.

Once the tomatoes look sweet and inviting, crack the eggs over each tomato-heaped toast and drizzle a little yoghurt over each one. Scatter the spring onions and chilli flakes over. Bake for 5–10 minutes, or until the eggs are set, and serve.

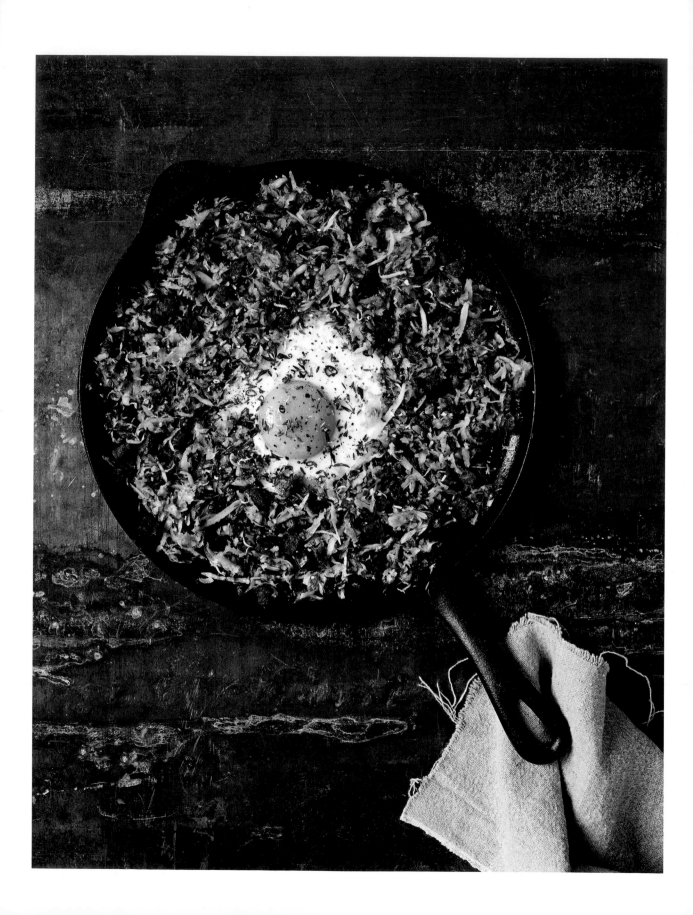

PARSNIP CHORIZO HASH WITH LIME, THYME AND FRIED EGGS

 2 PORTIONS
PER SERVING

PREP   10 MINS
COOK   20 MINS
SERVES 4

a few glosses of olive oil

2 onions, finely chopped

150g chorizo (cooking or cured), cut or broken into small pieces

½ tsp cumin seeds, plus a little extra to garnish (optional)

500g parsnips, coarsely grated

2 garlic cloves, finely chopped

grated zest and juice of 1 lime

4 fresh thyme sprigs, leaves only

4 eggs

a pinch of chilli flakes or chilli powder (optional)

sea salt and freshly ground black pepper

Heat a large frying pan and add a gloss of olive oil. Tumble in the onions and cook over a medium-low heat until glossy and tender.

Crank up the heat and add the chorizo to the pan. Sizzle until the fat renders out a bit and the chorizo is golden, 5–10 minutes.

Toss in the cumin seeds, parsnips, garlic and a hit of pepper. Add an extra gloss of oil, if needed. Fry over a medium-high heat, stirring occasionally, until the parsnips are tender and starting to colour a little around the edges.

Add a good hit of lime zest and juice. Scatter the thyme leaves over, saving a few to garnish. Season to taste, and add a little more lime, as needed.

Make 4 little indentations in the pan for your eggs. Add a little oil in each space and crack your eggs into the centre of each. Pop a lid on, if you wish, to help the eggs set on top.

Once cooked to your liking, scoop each egg, along with a surrounding nest of hash (and any stray bits) onto a plate. Finish with a pinch of salt, cumin seeds, thyme leaves and chilli flakes or powder.

Variation: for a vegetarian option, instead of the chorizo, add 1 tsp smoked sweet paprika and a pinch of chilli powder when you add the parsnips and cumin. Scatter salted, chopped Marcona almonds (or normal almonds) over just before serving. This is lovely with avocado slices on the side.

PUMPKIN, CHILLI AND HALLOUMI FRITTATA

 PORTIONS PER SERVING 1.5

PREP   10 MINS
COOK   30 MINS
SERVES   4

a few glosses of olive or rapeseed oil

175–200g halloumi cheese, sliced

500g pumpkin or butternut or autumnal squash, peeled and cut into bite-sized chunks

2 red chillies, finely chopped

1 garlic clove, finely chopped

2 tsp cider or white wine vinegar

1 tsp runny honey

1 small bunch of fresh mint or thyme, roughly chopped

6 eggs, beaten

Heat the oven grill to high. If you don't have access to a grill, preheat the oven to 200°C/Gas 6, but make sure one of the oven shelves is set high up.

Heat a large frying pan and add a thin gloss of oil. Add the halloumi slices and cook over a medium heat until golden on each side, about 5 minutes, then remove from the pan and set aside.

Add a fresh gloss of oil to the pan. Cook the squash until soft and starting to colour, about 15 minutes.

Mix the chilli, garlic, vinegar and honey in a small dish. The aim is to make a sweet chilli sauce to glaze the squash. Taste, and add more chilli, honey or vinegar to your liking.

Once the squash is golden and tender, add the chilli sauce to the pan and fold through. Return the halloumi to the pan, dotting it and the squash evenly around the pan. Scatter over the mint or thyme and pour on the eggs.

Cook until the base is set, about 5 minutes, then flash under the grill or place in the oven for 5–10 minutes until puffed up and golden. Serve warm or at room temperature. Any leftovers will keep in the fridge for a day or two.

GRIDDLED AUBERGINES WITH FRIED EGG, CHILLI YOGHURT, WALNUTS AND MINT

 PORTION PER SERVING

PREP 10 MINS
COOK 20 MINS
SERVES 4

2 aubergines

a few glosses of olive oil

1 lemon (optional)

4 pita breads

4 eggs

100ml natural or Greek yoghurt

1–2 tsp chilli flakes or 1 tbsp harissa (more or less to taste)

1 tsp smoked (sweet) paprika

a handful of fresh mint leaves

a handful of roughly chopped walnuts, toasted

sea salt and freshly ground black pepper

Slice the aubergines into 1cm-thick slices. Arrange in a single layer and sprinkle with a little salt and pepper.

Heat a large frying pan until smoking hot. You don't need any oil at this stage – I always find the aubergines lap it up and end up as oil sponges. Add the aubergine slices, again in a single layer (you may have to cook in batches or use two large pans). Cook until nicely charred, about 5 minutes on each side. This way you get a really intense, smoky flavour and a great texture. Grate a little lemon zest and squeeze a hit of juice over at the end, if desired, and gloss the slices with a little oil.

Toast the pita breads. Remove the aubergines from the pan and carefully slot them into the pitas (or serve the pitas on the side, or omit entirely if you're wheat/gluten-free).

Add a little oil to the frying pan. Crack the eggs into the pan, keeping them separate. Pop a lid on to help them set on top. Cook to your liking, or flip for 'over easy' eggs.

Tuck an egg into each aubergine-filled pita or perch it on top of a stack of cooked aubergines. Finish with a few dollops of yoghurt, along with a hit of chilli or harissa, a dusting of smoked paprika, a scattering of mint leaves and enough chopped walnuts to add a little texture and crunch.

Variation. Serve with 4 cherry tomatoes or a glass of fresh orange juice to bump this up to 2 servings.

Sundaes

THE BASICS: These are a fun way of getting kids into the kitchen. I lay out toppings like nuts, seeds, dried and fresh fruits, honey and jam, and let the children make their own creations with yoghurt and cereal. While I've included weights, I'd never bother getting the scales and measuring spoons out for these. Just throw together and make sure you pack in lots of fruit.

BANANA PEANUT BUTTER CUP

 1 PORTION
PER SUNDAE

PREP 10 MINS
COOK 5 MINS
SERVES 1

100g natural yoghurt

2 tsp peanut butter

½ tsp runny honey

a pinch of ground cinnamon

2 tbsp rolled oats

1 tsp cocoa powder

1 banana, thinly sliced

Mix the yoghurt, peanut butter, honey and cinnamon until well combined.

Toast the oats in a dry frying pan for a moment, if desired; toasting gives them a nuttier flavour. Add the cacao nibs or cocoa powder.

Layer up half the yoghurt, followed by half the oats (saving a pinch to scatter over the top) and half the banana slices. Repeat, finishing with the reserved oats.

PERSIAN PEAR

 1 PORTION
PER SUNDAE

PREP 10 MINS
COOK 5 MINS
SERVES 1

1 ripe pear •

100g Greek yoghurt

½ tsp rose water (optional)

a pinch of ground cardamom

2 tbsp rolled oats

1 tbsp crushed pistachios

a drizzle of honey

Peel, dice and core the pears, set aside. Mix the yoghurt with the rose water and cardamom.

Toast the oats and pistachios in a dry frying pan for a moment, if desired; toasting gives them a nuttier flavour.

Spoon half the yoghurt in your glass. Top with half the pistachio oats (bar a pinch for the top), followed by half the pear. Repeat, finishing with the reserved oats and a gloss of honey.

> ● *Stone fruit (for example peaches, nectarines, apricots) are a lovely summery substitute.*

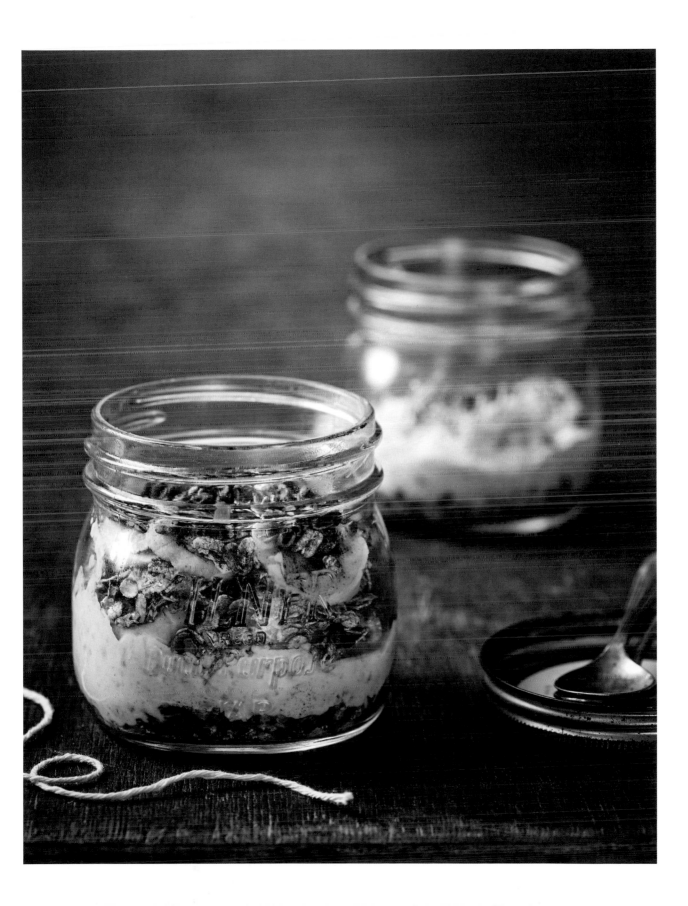

STRAWBERRY CHEESECAKE

 1.5 PORTIONS
PER SUNDAE

PREP   10 MINS
COOK   5 MINS
SERVES 1

120g fresh strawberries, hulled and roughly chopped●

½–1 tsp sugar or runny honey

100g vanilla yoghurt, or 100g natural yoghurt mixed with ½ tsp vanilla extract or ¼ of a pod vanilla seeds

2 tbsp cream cheese, curd cheese or mascarpone

2 tbsp rolled oats

1 heaped tbsp flaked or roughly chopped almonds

In a bowl, mix the strawberries with the sugar or honey, stirring until all the juices start to come out of the strawberries, creating a luscious sauce. In a separate bowl, whip the yoghurt and cheese together.

Toast the oats and almonds in a dry frying pan over a medium heat until the almonds are golden.

Spoon half the oats and almonds into the bottom of a glass. Pour in some of the strawberry juices and top with half the yoghurt, followed by half the strawberries. Repeat.

● *Or use any summer fruit. Cherries make a delicious alternative.*

PIÑA COLADA

1.5 PORTIONS
PER SUNDAE

PREP   10 MINS
COOK   5 MINS
SERVES 1

1 tbsp cashews

1 tbsp coconut flakes or desiccated coconut

1 tbsp rolled oats

a pinch of ground allspice (optional)

100g natural or coconut yoghurt (or 100g natural yoghurt mixed with 2 tbsp coconut milk)

120g fresh pineapple, cut into smallish cubes

Toast the cashews in a dry frying pan over a medium heat, and when just about golden add the coconut. Toast until fragrant and flecked with hints of golden brown. Stir in the oats and allspice, if using. Toast for a moment longer.

Layer up half the yoghurt, followed by half the nutty oats (saving a pinch to scatter over the top) and half the pineapple in a glass. Repeat, finishing with the reserved nutty oats.

Fruit Shakes

THE BASICS: You can use pretty much any recipe in the Breakfast chapter as a launchpad for a shake. The Morning Mojito (see page 46) can be blitzed up with a trickle of apple juice to make a fantastic smoothie. You can also treat the breakfast truffles are like an instant smoothie bomb: just drop into a blender with a splash of yoghurt or coconut milk and juice. The key to making a really luscious smoothie is temperature. Chill your ingredients first, use frozen fruit or shake the final drink with ice.

ORCHARD SHAKE

 PORTIONS PER SHAKE

PREP	5 MINS
COOK	NIL
SERVES	1

2 ripe and juicy plums •

150ml apple juice

a pinch of fresh lavender flowers or leaves

Simply whizz all the ingredients together with a hand blender, a traditional blender or in a food processor until smooth. Drink cold. Can be made the night before if kept in the fridge.

● *No plums? Swap with any other ripe and juicy stone fruit: ½ a peach or nectarine, or 40g sweet cherries.*

LAZY ENGLISH GARDEN

I'm a lazy gardener and a lazy cook, and I know I'm not alone. This smoothie was inspired by laid-back approaches. It's full of things that are effortless to grow, and it's a green drink, full of healthy vitamins, that doesn't require a juicer. If you do have a juicer and aren't feeling lazy, you could press your own apple juice, but at least the lazy option is there.

 PORTIONS PER SMOOTHIE

PREP	10 MINS
COOK	NIL
SERVES	1

50g frozen apple, diced

50g fresh spinach, roughly chopped (the finer, the better)

a few fresh mint leaves

200ml apple juice

Tumble the frozen apple hunks into a food processor or tall dish suitable for hand-blending. Add the spinach, mint and juice and whizz with a hand blender, a traditional blender or in a food processor until smooth.

NOTE: Apples freeze beautifully. Just peel, cut into hunks and toss with a little lemon juice to stop them browning. Tuck into a freezer-proof container and store for up to a year.

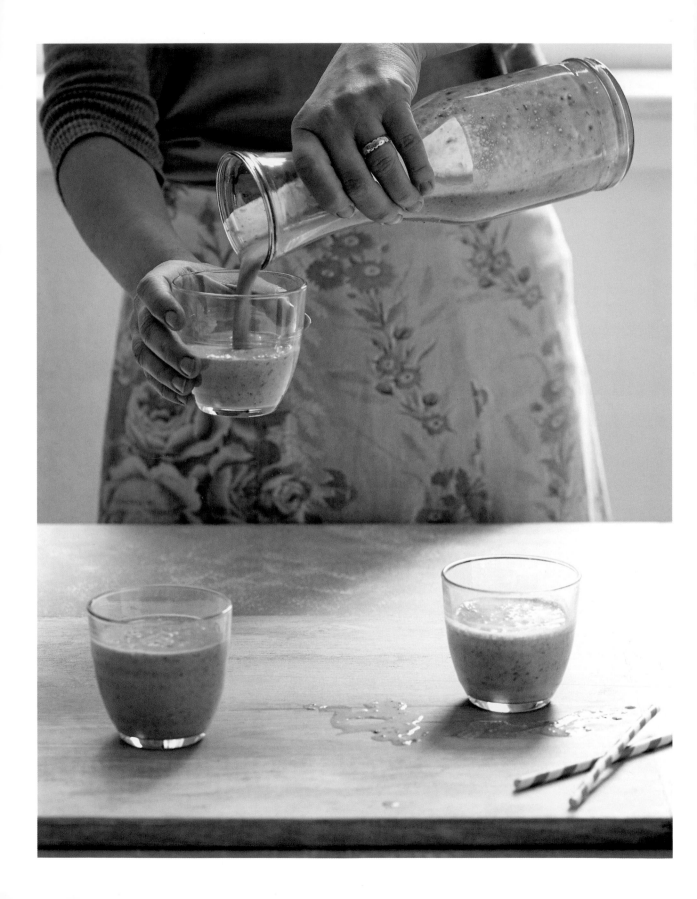

STRAWBERRY COCONUT SHAKE

For best results, refrigerate your coconut milk before whizzing up. This will give you a nice cold smoothie. But, keep your strawberries at room temperature, if possible, as the fridge tends to dull the sweetness. Out of season, however, opt for frozen strawberries.

**PORTION
PER SERVING**

PREP   5 MINS
COOK   NIL
SERVES 4

400g fresh strawberries, tops trimmed off

400ml coconut milk

1 tsp vanilla extract or seeds scraped from 1 pod (optional)

2 tbsp runny honey, coconut blossom sugar or your favourite sweetener, to taste

Blend the strawberries, coconut milk and vanilla together with a hand blender, a traditional blender or in a food processor until smooth. Whizz in a little honey or sweetener, if needed, to taste.

Divide between glasses or chill until ready to serve.

A COFFEE DATE

**PORTIONS
PER SMOOTHIE**

PREP   5 MINS
COOK   NIL
SERVES 1

1½ frozen bananas, chopped

1½ dates, stoned and chopped

seeds from 2 cardamom pods, finely ground (optional)

100ml almond milk (or cow's milk, soy, coconut)

100ml strong freshly brewed coffee (warm or cold) •

Blitz all the ingredients with a hand blender, traditional blender or in a food processor until smooth. Drink straight away.

● *If you're avoiding caffeine, try strongly brewed chicory coffee. It's delicious in this shake.*

INSTANT ALMOND MILK
Whizz 35g ground almonds (or grind your own almonds or other nuts first) with 65ml water.

KERALAN SUNRISE

I got the idea of putting turmeric in a smoothie from an LA juice bar, The Punchbowl. They come up with the most incredible flavour combinations, like the lovely Rita Hayworth: strawberries, rose water and primrose oil. I also love the brilliantly named Greeña Colada, featuring kale, coconut water, avocado, pineapple and lime.

They also feature mango with turmeric on the menu. This is my ridiculously simple take on it. I would normally pair mango with cardamom, or even a pinch of saffron, but this works just as well. If you stumble upon fresh turmeric, nab some. It looks like mini fresh ginger and can be used in the same way.

 PORTIONS PER SERVING

PREP   10 MINS
COOK   NIL
SERVES 1

150g fresh and ripe or frozen mango

75ml coconut milk

50ml water

a pinch of ground turmeric (I add about ⅛ tsp, but start with a little and increase to taste)

a hint of honey, maple syrup or your favourite sweetener

Pop the mango, coconut milk and water into a food processor or blender and whizz until smooth.

Add a hint of turmeric, to taste, and whizz in a little more water if it's too thick for your liking. Finally, add a little honey or similar sweetener, to taste.

Serve immediately. Freeze any leftovers as ice lollies.

Breakfast Truffles

THE BASICS: These are ridiculously easy to make and they're a fun way to pack in a portion of fruit. They're delicious for breakfast with fresh fruit or a smoothie, and also go down a treat in children's lunchboxes. For adults, they're a great substitute for a mid-morning biscuit.

If you don't have a food processor, just tip everything onto a large cutting board and chop finely with a large knife. Toss in a bowl and squeeze the medley together with your hands. If going down this route, you may need to add a little extra oil or juice to the mix.

LEMON, PRUNE AND ALMOND

 PORTION PER
2 TRUFFLES

PREP	10 MINS (PLUS OVERNIGHT SOAKING)
COOK	NIL
MAKES	12

100g pitted prunes, soaked overnight*

100g rolled oats

100g finely chopped almonds, toasted

1 tsp vanilla extract or seeds from ¼ of a pod

½ tsp ground cinnamon

zest and juice of 1 lemon (4–6 tbsp)

1–2 tbsp olive, almond or coconut oil, if needed

Drain your soaking prunes. Tip the prunes, oats, half of the almonds, the vanilla and the cinnamon into a food processor. Add the lemon zest and 4 tbsp of lemon juice. Blitz until the mix comes together into a ball. Trickle more lemon juice and/or a little oil into the mix, if it's looking too dry. If it's too wet, add more oats.

Roll into a log, then divide into 12 evenly sized pieces.

Shape into balls. Roll the balls into the remaining almonds to coat. To help the almonds stick, roll the balls in a little dish of water first. These will keep in the fridge for a week.

● *Forgot to soak overnight? Just simmer your prunes in enough water to cover for 5–10 minutes, or until just tender.*

DATE, ORANGE AND SESAME

 PORTION PER
2 TRUFFLES

PREP	10 MINS
COOK	NIL
MAKES	12

100g pitted dates, roughly chopped

100g rolled oats

100g sesame seeds, toasted

½ tsp ground cinnamon

¼ tsp ground ginger

a grating of orange zest (optional)

4–5 tbsp orange juice

Tip the dates, oats, half the sesame seeds and the cinnamon, ginger and a little orange zest, if using, into a food processor. Add the orange juice. Blitz until the mix comes together into a ball. Add a little more juice if the mix is looking too dry. If it's too wet, add more oats.

Roll into a log, then divide into 12 evenly sized pieces.

Shape into balls. Roll in the remaining sesame seeds to coat and serve. These will keep in the fridge for a week.

FIG, ROSE AND COCONUT

1 **PORTION PER**
2 TRUFFLES

PREP	10 MINS
COOK	NIL
MAKES	12

100g dried figs, roughly chopped

100g rolled oats

100g desiccated coconut, toasted if desired

1–2 tsp rose water

4 tbsp coconut oil

Tip the dried figs, oats, half the desiccated coconut and a teaspoon of the rose water into a food processor. Add the coconut oil. Blitz until the mix comes together into a ball. Add a little more oil if the mix is looking too dry. If it's too wet, add more oats.

Taste. Trickle in more rose water, if needed.

Roll into a log, then divide into 12 evenly sized pieces.

Shape into balls. Roll the balls in the remaining desiccated coconut to coat and serve. These will keep in the fridge for a week.

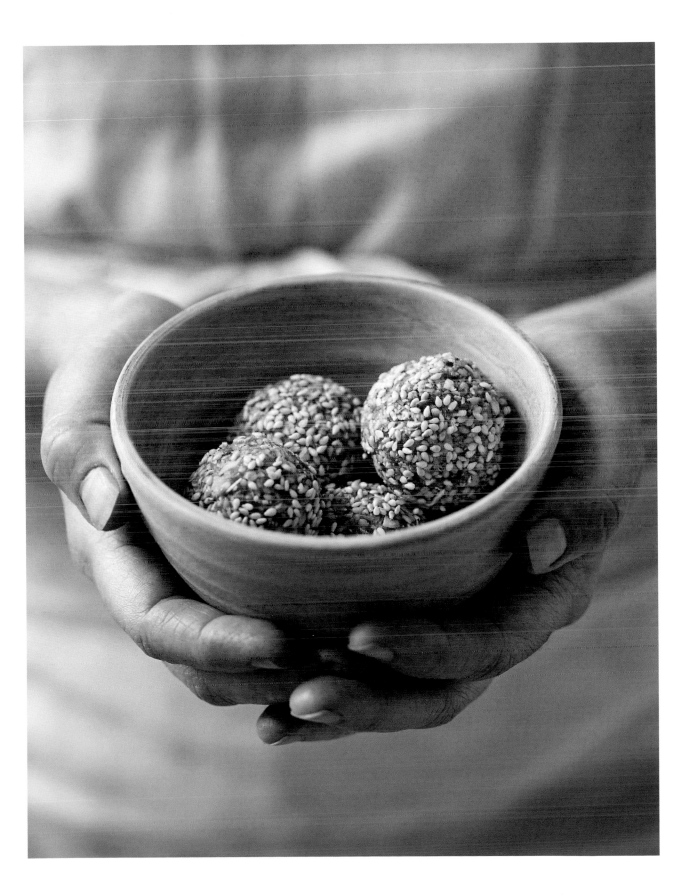

APRICOT, CARDAMOM AND CASHEW

 1 PORTION PER 2 TRUFFLES

PREP   10 MINS
COOK   NIL
MAKES   12

100g dried apricots, roughly chopped

100g rolled oats

100g cashews, raw or toasted

seeds from 6 cardamom pods, crushed

1 tbsp coconut or extra virgin olive oil

4 tbsp apple or orange juice

Tip the apricots, oats, half of the cashews, and the cardamom seeds into a food processor. Add the oil and apple or orange juice. Blitz until the mix comes together into a ball. Add a little more juice if the mix is looking too dry. If it's too wet, add more oats.

Roll into a log, then divide into 12 evenly sized pieces.

Chop the remaining cashew nuts as finely as possible. Shape into balls. Roll the balls in the chopped nuts to coat. To help the chopped cashews stick, roll the balls in a little dish of water first. These will keep in the fridge for a week.

RAISIN, APPLE AND HAZELNUT

 1 PORTION PER 2 TRUFFLES

PREP   10 MINS
COOK   5 MINS
MAKES   12

100g raisins

100g rolled oats

100g hazelnuts, finely chopped or crushed, (toasted if desired)

½ tsp ground cinnamon

4–5 tbsp apple juice

Tip the raisins, oats, half the hazelnuts and the cinnamon into a food processor. Add the apple juice. Blitz until the mix comes together into a ball. Add a little more juice if the mix is looking too dry. If it's too wet, add more oats.

Roll into a log, then divide into 12 evenly sized pieces.

Shape into balls. Roll the balls in the remaining hazelnuts to coat and serve. These will keep in the fridge for a week.

Fruit Salads

THE BASICS: Let's face it, fruit salads can be boring. There's so much to offer beyond the standard apple, grape and melon combos you see in supermarkets. All it takes is a scattering of herbs or spices, or maybe some crunchy and sticky honey-toasted nuts. Toast crumbs, perhaps. Then you've got something worth getting out of bed for.

CRUNCHY THINGS ON TOP: Go bananas with nuts. Adding a crunchy protein hit to your fruity salad not only makes it more substantial, it gives it texture and visual glitz. Seeds also add crunch and look the part. It doesn't stop there. You could try brioche or croissant croutons.

SPICE IT UP: Get out all those spices you never use and dash them on some fruit. Try Szechuan peppercorns on strawberries; fennel seeds on pineapple; cloves with oranges; peach and cardamom; apple and a little ground star anise; apricots and ginger.

COCKTAIL CREATIONS: Turn your favourite cocktail into a fruit salad (without the booze, of course – well, unless appropriate). A piña colada fruit salad would be a hit: pineapple, flakes of fresh or toasted coconut and bananas, finished off with lime zest, juice and some toasted cashews, with a hint of sea salt.

HERBACEOUS: Venture beyond mint and try basil with orange; lemon verbena with berries; lemon thyme with quince; rosemary with peaches.

TEMPERATURE: Who says a fruit salad has to be cold? Hot fruit is fun. A roasted peach fruit salad with toasted pine nuts, a gloss of saffron-infused honey and a wedge of cold ricotta gives the humble fruit salad a whole new raison d'être.

APPLE SLAW WITH DATES AND LEMON

2 PORTIONS
PER SERVING

PREP   15 MINS
COOK   5 MINS
SERVES 4

4 apples

zest of 1 lemon, plus a good
  squeeze of juice

8 dates

4 tbsp almonds, crushed or
  chopped

Coarsely grate the apples, leaving the skin on for added texture and colour. Add the lemon zest and juice and mix through. Stone and thinly slice the dates and fold through.

Toast the almonds in a dry frying pan over a medium heat, and scatter over the top.

SUMMER BERRY CRUSH

 2 PORTIONS
PER SERVING

PREP   10 MINS
COOK   NIL
SERVES 4

600g summer berries and
currants (strawberries,
raspberries, blueberries,
blackberries, blackcurrants,
redcurrants)

1–2 tsp sugar (any kind)

a hit of spice or herbs ●

Rinse the fruit. Dust with sugar, starting with 1 teaspoon. Give them a good scrunch with your hands to get their juices flowing.

Add your chosen spice or herbs and mix through, breaking the bigger pieces of fruit up by squeezing it between your fingers (this bit's fun), or if you don't want to get your hands messy, crush with a fork. Taste. Add a little more sugar, spice and/or herbs, as needed.

> ● *Vanilla's the classic, and for a reason. Scrape in the seeds from ½ a pod or use 1 tsp extract. Beautiful capped with a wedge of creamy ricotta.*
>
> *Chinese five spice is a complete head turner. I tried this salad with every jar of spice in my cupboard and this was the winner.*
>
> *Rose water. Just use a drop (no more than 1 tsp). This works particularly well with the red fruits. Finish with thick Greek yoghurt and fresh (non-sprayed) rose petals.*
>
> *Fresh mint is another classic. Stack 5 bigger leaves on top of one another, roll up and thinly slice. Finish with smaller mint leaves.*
>
> *Lemon verbena is the most adored herb in my garden. Use it like mint, chopping a few of the bigger leaves and scattering a few smaller leaves on top.*

HOT CROSS FRUIT SALAD

2 PORTIONS
PER SERVING

PREP   15 MINS
COOK   5 MINS
SERVES 4

1 heaped tbsp currants or
raisins

8 oranges or 10–12
clementines

½ tsp mixed spice

3 tbsp flaked almonds

3 tbsp toast crumbs

Place the currants or raisins in a mug. Cover with boiling water, allowing them to plump up for 5–10 minutes.

Grate or use a zester to gather a good pinch of orange or clementine zest. Scrape into a little dish and set aside. Slice off the top and bottom of each orange, so they stand on a cutting board. Carve the skin off the sides so the orange is fully peeled, then cut into sunshiny rounds. Dust the zest and half of the mixed spice over the oranges. Squeeze any juice you can extract from the peel over the fruit.

Heat a little frying pan over a medium heat and add the almonds and toast crumbs. Toast until the almonds are just golden, then fold in the remaining mixed spice.

Drain the soaking dried fruit. Dot over the salad and scatter the spiced almond crumbs over the top.

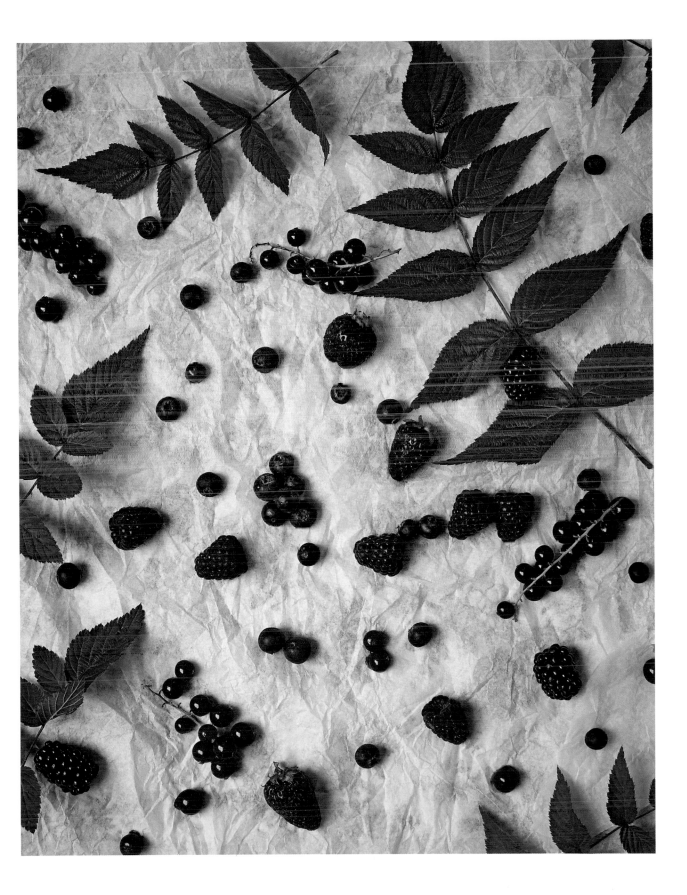

MORNING MOJITO

I'm probably taking some liberties here. This isn't a drink and it doesn't contain rum, but it's a good way to perk up a fruit salad, even without the alcohol. And if you really want to add some rum, I'm not going to stop you. In fact, as a pud, it's quite a novel way to end a meal. I'm wondering if Hemingway would approve? (Possibly not.)

 PORTIONS PER SERVING

PREP   15 MINS
COOK   NIL
SERVES 4

500g ripe mango•

a handful of fresh mint leaves

a sprinkling of sugar, to taste (optional)

zest of 1–2 limes, plus a good squeeze of juice

Peel and carve the cheeks off your mango. Slice each into a few strips. Carve the flesh from the skin and cut into slivers. Cut the flesh from around the stone of the mango, too, also cutting it into slivers.

Stack 10 mint leaves on top of each other. Roll them up and thinly slice. Mix the mint wisps with the mango and taste. If your mango's on the tangy side, sprinkle a little sugar over and mix through. Add the lime zest and juice, taste again, and add a little more sugar, if needed.

Finish with a scattering of small fresh mint leaves on top and serve.

> • *Mango is my favourite fruit to mingle mojito flavours with, but (in order of preference) the following fruits also work a treat: nectarine, pineapple, apple, strawberries and melon.*

BANANA WITH HONEYED HAZELNUTS

 PORTION PER SERVING

PREP   10 MINS
COOK   5 MINS
SERVES 4

4 good-sized bananas or 6 smaller ones•

1 lemon (optional)

4 tbsp hazelnuts, crushed

1 tbsp runny honey, maple syrup or agave

a dollop of yoghurt, goat's curd, ricotta or crème fraîche, to serve

Peel and halve your bananas, then slice lengthwise. Or just cut into rounds, if you prefer. Add a hint of lemon zest and juice, if desired, to cut through the sweetness and to keep the bananas from browning.

Toast the hazelnuts in a dry frying pan over a medium heat. Once fragrant and toasty, swirl in the honey, syrup or agave until the nuts are nicely coated. Scatter over the bananas and serve on their own or with a dollop of yoghurt, goat's curd, ricotta or crème fraîche.

> • *Swap the fresh bananas for frozen. You can freeze bananas whole in a plastic tub. When ready to use, thinly slice at an angle and serve with the warm, honeyed nuts as above. It's wonderfully refreshing on a hot day.*

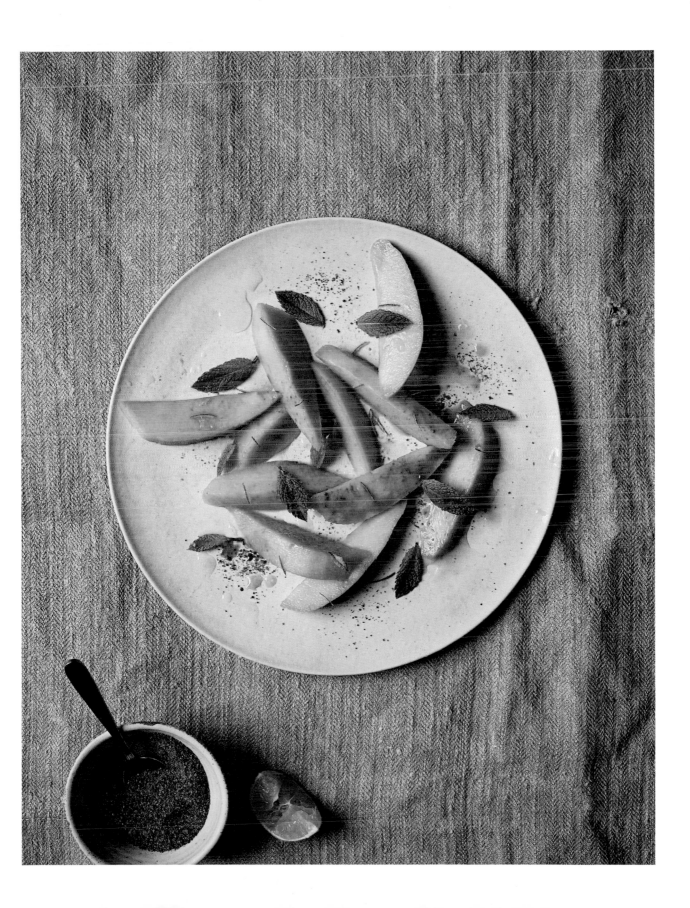

Hot Fruit

THE BASICS: Warming fruit totally transforms it. The simple act of applying a little heat reduces all those lovely juices within the fruit to sweet, sticky syrup. I can't think of a fruit that doesn't become irresistible after a little roasting or pan frying – even slices or segments of oranges or lemons become utterly phenomenal after a bit of oven bathing.

The following recipes are some of my favourite fruit transformations, but try their carriers with different fruits: top your blinis with slices of peaches sweetened with maple syrup; sizzle pitted cherries for your cacao-studded pancakes; roast whole fresh figs for your cinnamon toasts, or halved apricots for your honeyed toasts...

ROASTED PLUMS ON CINNAMON TOASTS

 PORTION PER SERVING

PREP 15 MINS
COOK 35 MINS
SERVES 4

8 plump plums or
  12 smaller ones

4–8 slices of bread

enough butter, olive or nut
  oil to gloss the bread

2 tbsp sugar (any kind)

1 tsp ground cinnamon

a dollop of crème fraîche,
  yoghurt or mascarpone, to
  serve (optional)

Preheat the oven to 200°C/Gas 6.

Halve and stone the plums and arrange in a roasting tray. Cook for 30 minutes, or until tender and visibly sweet (they'll have shrunk and their juices will have cooked down into a sticky syrup).

As the plums cook, gloss the top side of your bread slices with butter or oil. Mix the sugar with the cinnamon and sprinkle over the toasts.

Whip the plums out of the oven once done. If you have a grill, switch to the grill setting; if not, the oven will do. Place your toasts in the oven, cinnamon sugar side up. Cook until golden on top, about 5–7 minutes. The aim is to caramelise the sugar so you have a lovely sweet crunchy top.

Arrange the toast on plates and pile your plums on top. Serve with a dollop of crème fraîche, yoghurt or mascarpone, if you like.

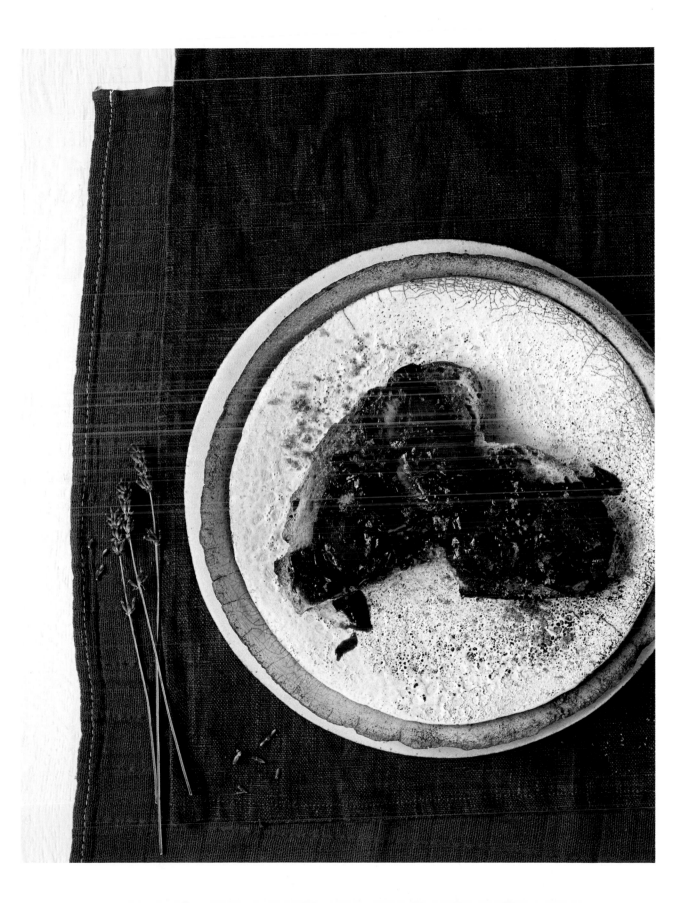

ROASTED APPLE WITH HONEYED NUTMEG TOASTS

 1 PORTION
PER SERVING

PREP   15 MINS
COOK   40 MINS
SERVES 4

4 good-sized apples

4–8 slices of bread from
your favourite loaf (a nutty
rye or spelt loaf works a
treat here)

a few slicks of butter

a generous gloss of honey

a good grating of nutmeg•

Preheat the oven to 200°C/Gas 6.

Core your apples. Set the apples on their sides and make a 1cm-deep incision around the apples' widest girth, as if giving them a belt. This gives them room to swell and keeps them from bursting their skins.

Place the apples in a roasting dish. Cook at the top of the oven until fully tender, about 30 minutes.

Gloss one side of each slice of bread with butter and honey. Grate a dusting of nutmeg over the top. Pop in the oven, again towards the top, and cook until crisp and just golden on top, about 5–10 minutes.

Transfer the apples to a plate. Pull off the top half of the skin. Gloss with a little honey if it's too tart. Cut the toasts into fingers or triangles. Dunk them into the apples or spoon onto the toast.

> • *No nutmeg? Just swap for your favourite spice, or let the honey do the talkin'.*

CARAMELISED PINEAPPLE AND DATES, YOGHURT AND SUNFLOWER SEEDS

 3 PORTIONS
PER SERVING

PREP   15 MINS
COOK   15 MINS
SERVES 4

a gloss of oil

8 fresh slices of pineapple
(2–3cm thick), peeled

2 star anise, crushed
(optional)

8 dates, halved and pitted

200g Greek yoghurt

2–3 tbsp sunflower seeds

Heat a large frying pan over a medium heat and add a gloss of oil.

Arrange the pineapple slices in the pan in a single layer; either cook in batches or use a second pan.

Dust a pinch of star anise over the pineapple, if using. Sizzle the slices until golden on both sides; it only takes a few minutes.

Once the pineapples are done, toss the dates in the pan and spoon through the residual oil and pineapple juices. You just want to gently warm them. Arrange the pineapple and dates on plates and add a dollop of yoghurt.

Tumble the seeds in your still-warm frying pan and toast until just golden. Scatter over the top of each plate and serve warm.

CACAO NIB PANCAKES WITH RASPBERRY SAUCE

 1.5 PORTIONS
PER SERVING

PREP 10 MINS
COOK 20 MINS
SERVES 4

FOR THE PANCAKES
2 eggs

225g wholegrain flour (rye, wheat, kamut, spelt)

1 tbsp baking powder

300ml orange or apple juice

1 tbsp olive or coconut oil, plus extra for cooking

1 tsp vanilla extract or seeds from ⅓ a vanilla pod

50g cacao nibs or chopped dark chocolate

a gloss of butter

FOR THE TOPPING
500g fresh raspberries•

100ml water

1 tbsp sugar (any kind), runny honey or maple syrup

vanilla yoghurt or mascarpone, to serve (optional)

Whisk the eggs until frothy. Add the remaining pancake ingredients and fold through until you have a smooth batter.

Place a large frying pan, or two smaller ones, over a medium-high heat. When the pan is hot, drizzle in a little oil and swirl around or use a pastry brush or cloth to spread it evenly; you just want a gloss.

Dollop 2 dessertspoons of batter for each pancake (make them smaller or larger, if you like) into the pan. Reduce the heat and cook the pancakes until you can see little bubbles working their way from the outside to the middle. Once they reach the centre, flip, and cook for a minute or two on the other side. Don't be tempted to press the pancakes into the pan as it will squash out all the air bubbles that make them light and fluffy.

Pile the warm pancakes on to plates. Gloss with butter. I like to arrange them side by side rather than in big stacks.

Rinse the pan and return to the hob over a high heat to make the topping. Add the berries and water and sizzle until the berries are softened, warm and juicy. If you have used a vanilla pod, toss it into the pan too. Lower the heat and swirl in your sweetener of choice. Let it cook into the sauce, then taste and adjust to your liking. Serve the warm berries over the pancakes, finished with a dollop of yoghurt or mascarpone, if using.

> • *No raspberries? Swap them for strawberries, pitted cherries, redcurrants or slices of ripe pear and warm with a little honey/sugar and water as above. Or just top with slices of fresh banana and a drizzle of honey or maple syrup.*

BLINIS WITH WARM BLUEBERRIES

 PORTIONS PER SERVING

PREP 10 MINS
COOK 20 MINS
SERVES 4

FOR THE BLINIS

2 eggs

175g buckwheat flour

1 tbsp baking powder

300ml apple juice

1 tsp vanilla extract

½ tsp ground cinnamon

2 tbsp oil (olive, coconut, rapeseed), plus extra for cooking

a gloss of butter

FOR THE TOPPING

500g blueberries•

100ml water

1 tbsp sugar, runny honey, maple syrup or your preferred sweetener

Whisk the eggs until frothy. Add the remaining blini ingredients, really whisking the batter to get some air bubbles in there. Buckwheat flour has no gluten so there's no risk of overworking it.

Place a large frying pan, or two smaller ones, over a medium-high heat. When the pan is hot, drizzle in a little oil and swirl around or use a pastry brush or cloth to spread it evenly; you just want a gloss.

Dollop a dessertspoon of batter for each blini (make them smaller or larger, if you like) into the pan. Reduce the heat and cook the blinis until you can see little bubbles working their way from the outside to the middle. Once they reach the centre, flip, and cook for a minute or two on the other side. Don't be tempted to press the blinis into the pan as it will squash out all the air bubbles that make them light and fluffy. Pile the warm blinis on a plate. Gloss with butter.

Rinse the pan and return to the hob over a high heat to make the topping. Add the berries and water and sizzle until the berries are softened, warm and juicy. If you have used a vanilla pod, toss it into the pan too. Lower the heat and swirl in your sweetener of choice. Let it cook into the sauce, then taste and adjust to your liking. Serve the warm berries over the blinis.

NOTE: Don't overcook the fruit. You're not after jam, rather warm, just-about-to-pop berries in a light syrup of sugar/honey, water and their own juices.

> • *When the blueberry season finishes, try with blackcurrants, blackberries, elderberries or any seasonal fruit that takes your fancy.*

BITE: GROW YOUR LUNCH

Nothing makes you look at a vegetable with utter fascination more than growing it yourself from seed. I'm completely new to the game and still a bit childlike with wonder, but I also know many seasoned gardeners who still get a thrill from pulling a home-grown carrot from the ground.

Five things you can grow without a garden:

Peas: From seed to pea in just 14 weeks. Dwarf varieties grow beautifully in a window box or other container. Soak the seeds before planting them, then push them 5cm into your compost. Water well. Let them lap up the sun, and when the compost looks dry, give it a good soaking. You should see shoots within two weeks. Once the peas produce flowers, add an organic liquid seaweed feed when watering. You only need a tiny amount – it'll say how much on the bottle. Nothing tastes more delicious than a freshly picked pea.

Cook: Summer Garden Pottage on page 142.

Carrots: From seed to carrot in just 12 weeks. Paris Market and other dwarf or round varieties are ideal for containers. The seeds are microscopic. Dot them in rows and then cover with 2cm compost. Space the seeds 4–5cm apart. Give them a good watering as soon as you've planted them, then let them lap up the sun. You should see shoots within 3 weeks. They're ready to harvest when you can see the rounded tops of the carrots swelling up from the compost. Keep them watered when the compost starts to look dry, and for best results add a little organic seaweed feed when watering once the shoots appear.

Cook: Roasted Carrot, Lemon and Almond Tagine on page 175.

Beetroot: From seed to beetroot in 12 weeks. Push the seeds 2–3 cm into your compost. Or arrange in rows (the more space you give them, the bigger they'll grow) and cover with a 2–3cm layer of compost. Water well. Place in a warm, sunny spot and keep them watered when the compost starts to look dry. Add a little seaweed feed to your water once the shoots have come up. As with carrots, you'll know they're ready when you can see the rounded tops swelling from the compost.

Cook: Beetroot, Orange and Poppy Slaw on page 88. Grow poppies alongside your beetroot and you'll have grown more than half the recipe.

Radishes: From seed to radish in just 6 weeks, or less for some varieties. Plant the seeds 2cm deep, allowing 3–4 cm around each seed. Water well. Place in a sunny spot and keep them nicely watered. Add a little seaweed feed to your water once the shoots have come up. You'll know they're ready when you can see the rounded tops swelling from the compost.

Cook: Radish and Tarragon Tzatziki on page 71. Pop some tarragon in the pot with the radishes and you've got the entire dip growing in the pot. It's a great dinner party trick to get your guests harvesting their own meal.

Tomatoes: From seed to tomato in 20 weeks. You can just pluck the seeds from a shop-bought tomato and put them straight into a pot. The odds of them growing are in your favour. Opt for cherry tomatoes if you're growing in containers. The larger the pot or container, the better they'll grow, but you can produce tomatoes from containers as small as a teacup – you just won't get much fruit. Plant 2cm deep. Water well and keep in a warm, sunny spot. Once you see shoots, add a little seaweed feed to your water.

Cook: Summer Tomato and Seed Penne on page 114.

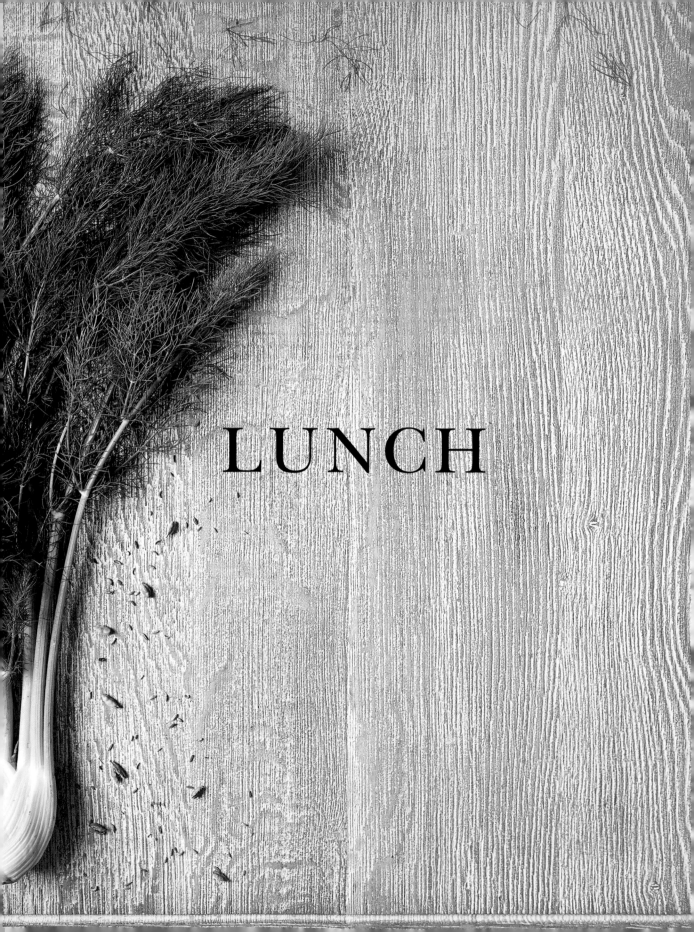

LUNCH

Soups and Stocks

THE BASICS: Soup is a great way to pack in the veg: on a cold day, warming, rich and inviting. My favourite soups are of the smooth and creamy variety; I've bumped all the thick, textured soups into the Fast chapter under Stews, where you can make more of a hearty meal of them. And I love little crunchy things sprinkled on top of soups, be they snippets of fried chorizo, salty toasted seeds or nuts, or fried breadcrumbs mixed with spice.

Homemade stock makes all the difference to soup, giving it a clean, pure flavour that stays true to the ingredients. My freezer is tiny and there's barely any room for me to be squirrelling away stocks in it. Instead, I keep a plastic tub in my fridge for all my veg odds and ends: half a carrot, the woody tops of a fennel bulb, odd celeriac trimmings, tough asparagus ends... When I need some stock, I blitz all these in my food processor, then fry off in oil with chopped onion and garlic, bay leaves and thyme sprigs until glossy. Toss in some parsley or carrot tops if you've got them, add water to cover then simmer for 10–15 minutes. Remove from the heat and leave to sit for a further 10 minutes. Strain and use straight away in your soup.

SUMMERY THAI MELON

This soup is ridiculously refreshing and outrageously delicious. The perfect light summer lunch or starter.

 1.5 PORTIONS PER
SERVING FOR 4

PREP 15 MINS
COOK NIL
SERVES 2–4

1 ripe galia or honeydew melon

1 cucumber

1 stalk of lemongrass

1 heaped tsp freshly grated ginger

a good pinch of finely chopped fresh chilli (more or less, to taste)

200ml coconut milk

a large handful of Thai or regular basil

a small handful of fresh mint

zest and juice of 1–2 limes

Halve the melon. Scoop out the seeds. Spoon the flesh from the skin straight into a blender or food processor.

Peel the cucumber. Roughly chop. Add with the melon.

Bash the lemongrass stalk until it flattens and softens a little. Peel the outer layer away. Thinly slice starting at the base. Finely chop until you have about 1 heaped teaspoon.

Add the lemongrass to the blender or food processor along with the ginger, chilli, coconut milk, basil, mint and the zest and juice of 1 of the limes.

Whizz until smooth. Taste. Add more lemongrass, ginger, chilli, herbs or lime juice as needed. Swirl in a bit more coconut milk, too, if needed. The balance really depends on the sweetness of your melon.

Once it's so good you can't stop eating it, pop it in the freezer to chill quickly or the fridge if you're serving it later. Lovely garnished with a swirl of coconut milk drizzled on top and some fresh basil leaves.

Variation: Swap the melon and cucumber for 160g fresh baby spinach. Up the coconut milk to 400ml, add a small garlic clove and a good pinch of sea salt to the mix. Blitz. Taste. Tweak. Serve cold and uncooked, or gently warmed.

MEXICAN ROAST PUMPKIN WITH LIME

This soup's an amazing way to transport your taste buds to sunnier climes when the weather turns cold. The sharp tang of the lime cuts through the sweetness of the squash beautifully. It's also packed full of vitamin C so is a great way to wave off a cold.

 3 PORTIONS
PER SERVING

PREP 10 MINS
COOK 45 MINS
SERVES 4

1kg squash or pumpkin

a gloss of olive oil

8 garlic cloves, left in their skins

½ fresh red chilli, finely chopped (or a good pinch of a soaked and finely chopped chipotle chilli) (more or less, to taste)

a large handful of fresh coriander, plus extra to garnish

a sprig of fresh mint, leaves only (optional), plus extra to garnish

zest and juice of 1 lime

1 litre hot veg stock

sea salt and freshly ground black pepper

Preheat oven to 220°C/Gas 7.

Quarter the squash and scoop out the seeds. Halve each quarter, rub with a little oil, salt and pepper, and pop the squash and garlic on a baking tray. Place in the oven, flesh-side up, on the top shelf (but not touching the top of the oven). Roast for 40 minutes.

Check the garlic cloves after 15 minutes (they'll cook faster than the squash). Remove them when they're squishy, but continue cooking the squash until all the excess moisture has cooked out and the flesh is soft enough to scoop from its skin. Scoop the flesh into the bowl of a blender or a food processor, or into a pot if you're planning to use a hand blender.

Pop the garlic cloves out of their skins. Add them to the squash along with the chilli, coriander, mint, if using, lime zest and juice, and a splash of the stock. Whizz, trickling in more stock until you've reached your desired consistency.

Garnish with fresh coriander and mint leaves.

BLACK BEAN AND SMOKED PEPPER

PORTIONS PER SERVING 3

PREP 10 MINS (LONGER IF USING FRESH RED PEPPER AND DRIED BLACK BEANS)

COOK 25 MINS

SERVES 4

a gloss of oil (olive, coconut, rapeseed)

2 onions, finely diced

2 garlic cloves, finely diced

2 tsp ground cumin

2 tsp smoked paprika

a pinch of chilli powder

4 piquillo peppers from a jar (often found in Spanish shops and delis), chopped ●

400g tin of chopped tomatoes

800g tins of black beans, drained ●●

500ml veg or chicken stock, warmed

a pinch of ground cinnamon and a grating of cacao or dark chocolate, to taste

dollops of crème fraîche, yoghurt or a crumble of feta, to serve

a handful of fresh coriander leaves, to serve

sea salt and freshly ground black pepper

Heat a large saucepan and add a gloss of oil. Tumble in the onions, add a pinch of salt and lower the heat, sizzling until tender.

Swirl in the garlic and spices. Cook for a moment, until fragrant. Fold in the red pepper and tomatoes and cook down a little until thickened. Add the beans and stock and simmer for 15 minutes to marry the flavours. Taste, season and adjust the spicing to your liking. Add a hint of cinnamon and/or cacao or dark chocolate.

Part blend the soup so it's a little chunky but also thick and a little creamy. Do this by sticking a hand blender into the pan and pulsing until the texture is right; or add half the soup to a blender or food processor, roughly purée, and tip back into the pot.

Garnish with dollops or crumbs of dairy (crème fraîche, yoghurt or feta) and fresh coriander leaves.

Serve the soup with the Seedy Avocado Toasts on page 84 to bump the veg up to 4 servings.

● *If you can't find these, swap for 2 small or 1 large red pepper roasted in a 200°C/gas 6 oven until so tender it collapses and the skin has blackened. Cool, whip the skin off, pluck out the stem and seeds and roughly chop.*

●● *Or use dried black turtle beans. Soak overnight with a pinch of bicarbonate of soda added to the water (this helps soften them). Drain and rinse, then boil in fresh, unsalted water until tender, about 1 hour. Drain and tumble into the soup as if they were drained beans from a tin. I find the texture greatly improved by cooking my own beans, but tinned ones are great for a quick fix.*

MOROCCAN BEETROOT WITH MINT LABNEH

The labneh needs to be made several hours before serving. Just mix a pinch of salt and your finely chopped mint leaves through the yoghurt. Tip the mixture out onto a large piece of muslin cloth or a clean, thin tea towel. Gather the corners of the muslin and tie up on the handle of a kitchen cupboard or somewhere similar, with a bowl set beneath it to catch the whey. It needs at least 4 hours' straining. Once done, scoop the thick minty yoghurt from the cloth and refrigerate until ready to serve (use the whey in place of milk or buttermilk in baking). If you want to skip this bit, just finish the soup with Greek yoghurt and fresh mint leaves.

 PORTIONS PER SERVING FOR 4

PREP   15 MINS (PLUS 4 HOURS STRAINING)
COOK   45 MINS
SERVES   4–6

1kg beetroot, peeled and cut into 3–4cm dice

2 onions, sliced

3 garlic cloves, peeled

a gloss of olive oil

2 tsp cumin seeds, toasted

1 tsp ground cinnamon

½ tsp ground coriander

½ tsp ground ginger

zest and juice of 1 orange or lime

2 sprigs of fresh mint leaves, finely chopped, plus extra leaves to garnish

1–1½ litres hot veg or chicken stock

sea salt and freshly ground black pepper

FOR THE LABNEH
a pinch of sea salt

4 sprigs of fresh mint, leaves finely chopped

500g natural yoghurt

Preheat the oven to 200°C/Gas 6. Place a large roasting tray in the oven to heat up.

Toss the beetroot, onion and garlic in a bowl. Add a pinch of salt and pepper and gloss with oil. Tumble onto the heated roasting tray and cook for 35 minutes or until fully tender.

Once tender and a little golden around the edges, fold the spices through the warm veg.

Tumble into a blender or food processor (or use a hand blender, tumbling everything into a pot). Add the zest and juice of the orange or lime, fresh mint and a trickle of stock. Blend. Continue blending, trickling the stock in little by little, until smooth and the consistency you like. If you gradually blend in the stock you should end up with a smooth and creamy soup. If it's still a little lumpy, slowly scrape through a fine mesh sieve until it is silky smooth. A bit of a pain but it does deliver a rather elegant soup.

Taste, and adjust the seasoning and spice until it is just right for you. Divide between bowls. Spoon a large tablespoon of labneh into the centre of each and garnish with a few mint leaves and a crack of black pepper.

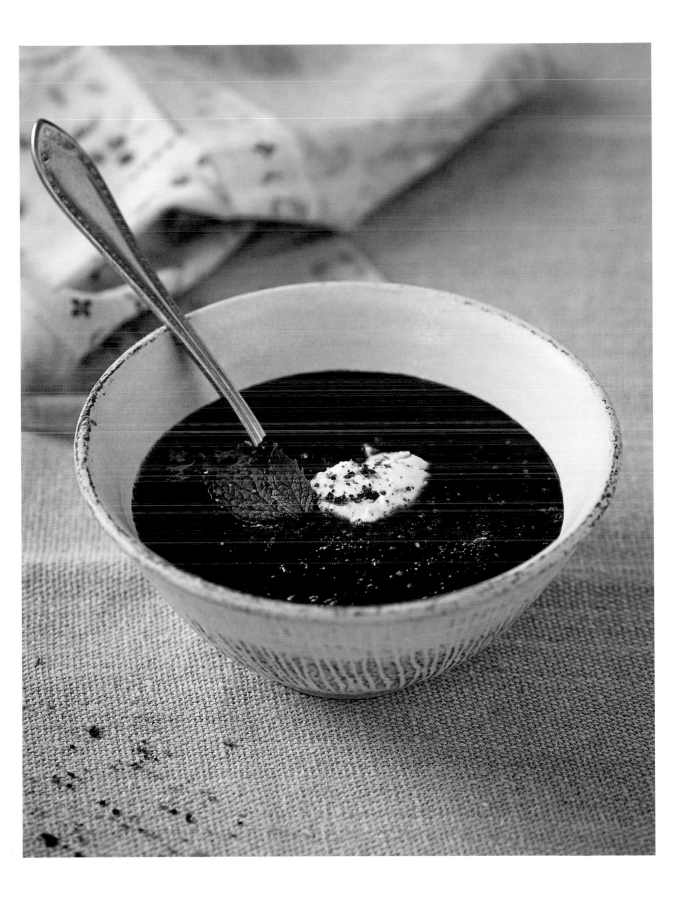

PARSNIP AND SHERRY MARMALADE BISQUE

My Catalan friend Demi invited a few of us over to share in a long, lazy Sunday lunch and I was tasked to bring the starter. I stumbled upon a gorgeous cauliflower salad with a Seville orange dressing from Jose Pizzaro, and was thinking of turning the combo into a soup along with some smoked Marcona almonds and sherry. I couldn't find cauliflower at the market, so plumped for parsnips instead and this soup was born. The combo of creamy parsnips and tangy marmalade with the smoky almonds is rather incredible.

 PORTIONS PER SERVING

PREP **20** MINS
COOK **30** MINS
SERVES **4**

500g parsnips, peeled and cut into chunks

a gloss of olive oil or a knob of butter

1 large onion, finely diced

2 bay leaves and/or 1 sprig fresh rosemary, finely minced

a handful of smoked or roasted Marcona almonds or toasted flaked almonds,

2 garlic cloves, finely minced

50ml olorosso or manzanilla sherry (optional)

2 tbsp marmalade•

500–750ml hot veg or chicken stock

250ml cow's, goat's or unsweetened almond milk

sea salt and freshly ground black pepper

Tumble the peeled parsnip chunks into a pan. Cover with water. Add a pinch of salt and boil until the parsnips are mashably tender.

Heat a frying pan. Add a gloss of oil or butter. Swirl your onions through with a pinch of salt and pepper. Add your bay and/or rosemary, if using. Cook over low heat until meltingly tender, about 15 minutes.

Drain the parsnips and return to the pan. Add the almonds.

As soon as the onions are soft, sweet and tender, remove the bay leaves, if using. Swirl in your garlic. Cook a moment, to soften. Add a slosh of sherry, if using. Let it reduce right down, until just 1–2 tablespoons remain. Swirl in the marmalade. If you're not using sherry, adding a little water or stock (or white wine) with the marmalade will help to loosen it up.

Add the sweet, sticky onions to your parsnips and almonds, along with a splash of stock. Blend in a food processor or blender or in the pan with a hand blender. Slowly trickle in the stock and milk until you reach your desired consistency.

Taste, season and tweak the sherry/marmalade/nut quantities as desired. Serve warm. This is lovely with a little swirl of marmalade (warmed and loosened with sherry or water) and a few almonds as a garnish.

> • *No marmalade? Use the zest and juice of 1 large or 2 small oranges and 1 tbsp runny honey instead. Let the juice and honey reduce down until sticky and thick.*

Little Salads

THE BASICS: This section is an homage to small medleys of lightly dressed raw veg that can be served up as sides or be paired with a bit of protein, be it grilled fish, fried halloumi, warm lentils or shreds of leftover roast lamb, to make a substantial main. These little salads are also brilliant for mezze or tapas-style feasts and parties, or simply mix one up for an easy light lunch. Wave bye-bye to boring lettuce and tomato and embrace a new realm of exciting fresh and salady possibilities.

SIMPLE SESAME CUCUMBER

This little salad is one of my all time favourite side dishes. Anytime I make something with a Japanese slant to it, I make this to go alongside. It's also a great snack or can make a simple lunch if you flake some smoked mackerel on top.

 1.5 PORTIONS
PER SERVING

PREP 10 MINS
COOK 5 MINS
SERVES 4

2 large cucumbers

a good pinch of sea salt

4 tbsp sesame seeds

Thinly slice the cucumbers. Dust a generous pinch of salt over. Mix through.

Get a large frying pan hot. Add the sesame seeds. Toast over medium-low heat until just golden.

Scatter the warm, toasted seeds over. Serve.

APPLE, CELERY AND CRUSHED PEANUT

PORTIONS PER SERVING

PREP 10 MINS
COOK 5 MINS
SERVES 4

4 large or 6 smaller apples

1 lemon

6 sticks of celery, thinly sliced, plus a few extra leaves

6 tbsp peanuts

200g natural yoghurt or goat's curd

1 tsp runny honey

a couple of pinches of sea salt

Thinly slice the apples horizontally, giving you pretty slices with a star pattern in the centre-most slices. Flick out any seeds. Grate the zest of the lemon over the apples and gloss them with a squeeze of juice. Scatter the celery slices and leaves over the apples. Gently mix them together in a pretty arrangement.

Heat a frying pan and add the peanuts, toasting them over a medium heat until fragrant and lightly coloured. Crush in a pestle and mortar, or in a bowl using the bottom of a glass or jar. Set aside.

Mix the yoghurt or goat's curd with the honey, a squeeze of lemon juice and a pinch of salt. Thin with a little cold water, if needed, and whisk until smooth.

Drizzle the dressing over the salad and finish with the crushed peanuts and a further pinch of sea salt, if desired.

BLOODY MARY

PORTIONS PER SERVING

PREP 15 MINS
COOK NIL
SERVES 4

1kg ripe tomatoes

1 garlic clove, finely chopped

a shake of cayenne pepper, chilli powder or Tabasco

1 tbsp Worcestershire sauce (or vegetarian equivalent)

4 sticks of celery, thinly sliced, plus celery leaves

a gloss of olive oil

zest and juice of 1 lemon

a scattering of fresh parsley

sea salt and freshly ground black pepper

Slice (larger toms) or halve (cherry toms) the tomatoes. Layer on a plate. Grate the garlic over. Dust with a pinch of salt, pepper, a hint of cayenne pepper, chilli powder or Tabasco and a shake of Worcestershire sauce. Scatter the celery over. Gently shuffle the ingredients together. Gloss the salad with a little olive oil.

Sprinkle over some lemon zest and a squeeze of juice. Taste. Adjust the seasoning and spice, as needed. I like to keep the salad on the milder side if I'm serving it to guests, laying all the accompaniments alongside the salad so they can tailor it to their heat tolerance. Finish with a scattering of parsley and/or celery leaves and a little more lemon zest.

Variation: this is also amazing with cold hard-boiled eggs, steak or grilled mackerel.

CAULIFLOWER COUSCOUS WITH CORIANDER AND ORANGE

I've made endless variations of this, adding blue cheese and walnuts, or Moroccan spices, dried fruit and nuts. This combo is one of my favourites as it celebrates a spice that I've rarely seen paired with cauliflower, and it works a treat.

 2.5 PORTIONS
PER SERVING

PREP 15 MINS
COOK 5 MINS
SERVES 4

1 head of cauliflower

4 oranges

a pinch of chilli powder

a gloss of olive oil

a large handful of fresh coriander or parsley leaves, chopped

1 tsp coriander seeds, toasted

4 tbsp sunflower seeds

4 tbsp pumpkin seeds

1 tbsp runny honey or maple syrup

sea salt and freshly ground black pepper

Carve the leaves and thick stalks from your cauliflower (use them in another dish; the leaves are gorgeous roasted with a little olive oil, sea salt and chilli flakes).

Pulse the cauliflower florets in a blender or food processor until they're finely chopped and couscous-like. If you haven't got a food processor, just chop the florets with a large knife until they're as fine as you can get them.

Scrape the cauli couscous into a bowl or serving dish. Grate the zest of 1 or 2 of the oranges into the couscous. Season with a pinch of salt, pepper and a hint of chilli powder, if using. Trickle a gloss of olive oil over the couscous.

Cut a slice off the tops and bottoms of your oranges. Carve the peel off the oranges and squeeze the juice from the cut peel over the couscous. Cut the oranges into segments, avoiding the fleshy membrane on the edge of each segment. Tumble the segments into the couscous, along with the coriander or parsley leaves and the coriander seeds.

Heat a little frying pan and tumble the sunflower and pumpkin seeds into the pan. Toast over a medium heat until fragrant and just golden, then take off the heat and swirl in the honey or maple syrup. Once the seeds are coated, scrape them from the pan onto your couscous.

SASSY CHERRY AND WATERCRESS SALAD WITH CRUSHED PISTACHIOS

2 PORTIONS PER SERVING

PREP 10 MINS
COOK NIL
SERVES 4

500g cherries

1 tsp runny honey, agave or sweetener of choice (optional)

1–2 tsp ras el hanout

1 tbsp olive oil, plus extra for glossing

150g watercress

a large handful of fresh mint leaves

a pinch of sea salt

a large handful of pistachios, shelled

Remove the stones and stems from the cherries – do this over a bowl so you catch all the juices. Add the cherries to the bowl and fold in the honey/sweetener. Add 1 teaspoon of the ras el hanout and the olive oil. Give everything a good squidgy mix using your hands, massaging the spices into the cherries.

Rinse the watercress leaves, shake dry and pile them on top. Add the mint and mix everything through. Taste, and add more spice, a little salt and more mint, as needed. Pile on plates and trickle a finishing gloss of olive oil over the top.

Lightly crush the pistachios in a pestle and mortar, or in a bowl using the base of a glass or jam jar. Scatter over the salad and serve.

A beautiful starter for a Moroccan feast, or pair with roasted duck for a summer supper.

RAS EL HANOUT
In a hot frying pan, toast 1 tsp coriander seeds, 1 tsp cumin seeds, 1 tsp black or pink peppercorns, 4 whole cloves and the seeds from 3 cardamom pods until fragrant. Grind the toasted spices in a pestle and mortar or in a metal bowl using the bottom of a glass or jam jar. Crush in a pinch of edible rose petals, if you have them. Mix in 1 tsp ground ginger, 1 tsp ground cinnamon, ¼ tsp ground nutmeg, ¼ tsp paprika and ¼ tsp ground allspice. Taste, and adjust the spice balance to suit. No two ras el hanout blends are the same, as the point is to make a fragrant mix of your choice. Sweet earthy spices form a large part, but you can up the spiciness with more pepper or a little chilli if you like.

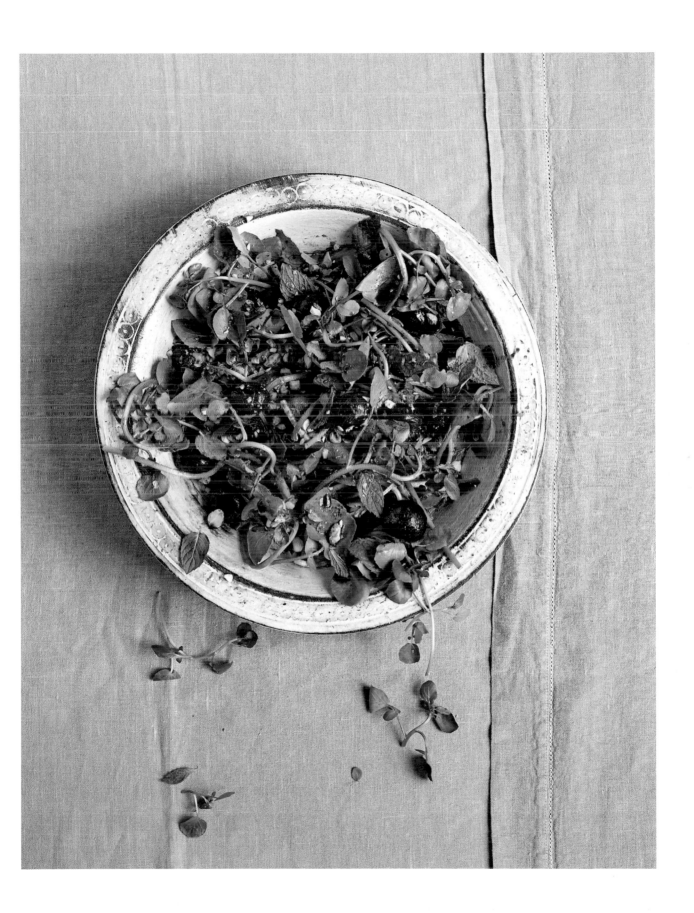

Dressings

THE BASICS: The fastest way to make a lettuce disappear is to marry it with a wicked little salad dressing. But dressings aren't just for glossing leaves; they also make brilliant dips for a mountain of veg.

The key to making a beautiful salad dressing is getting that balance between fat and acidity just right. I normally aim for a 50: 50 ratio. One of my favourite dressings is 4 tbsp olive oil shaken or stirred with 4 tbsp orange or lemon juice. You can then blend in herbs or shake in spices. Freshly grated ginger is a dream, and with lemon as your star it makes a pretty dressing for a simple avocado salad, with some fresh coriander.

There's a heap of scope beyond olive oil where fat is concerned. Use any oil, including melted coconut oil, a nut or seed butter, dairy, or whipped avocado as part of your fat ratio. The Zingy Tahini Dress and Creamy Coriander Dress offer some examples.

As far as acidity goes, there's vinegar and citrus fruits like lemon, lime and the entire orange family, from clementines to kumquat. These baby citrus fruits are gorgeous whizzed up (the whole fruit, skin and all) with olive oil, a little honey, salt and a pinch of Chinese five spice in a blender or food processor until creamy and delicious. Sieve out the skins and pips and you have an unforgettable dressing.

THE CREAMY CORIANDER

 PORTION FOR EVERY
80G OF SALAD DRESSED
OR VEG DIPPED

PREP 10 MINS
COOK NIL
SERVES 4

4 tbsp crème fraîche

1 tbsp olive oil

2 tsp Dijon mustard

1 tsp white wine vinegar or
   runny honey

1 tsp ground coriander
   (toasted whole seeds,
   then freshly ground,
   if possible)

sea salt and freshly ground
   black pepper

Place all the ingredients in a little bowl or jam jar and whisk together. Taste, and tweak the seasoning as needed, adding more mustard, cider, spice, crème fraîche, etc, until it's so good you could eat it on its own. Will keep in the fridge for 3–4 days.

Perfect with crispy, crunchy, refreshing veg like fennel, cucumber and wedges of baby gem or similar lettuces. It also makes a lovely marinade for aubergines (sliced or diced) before grilling.

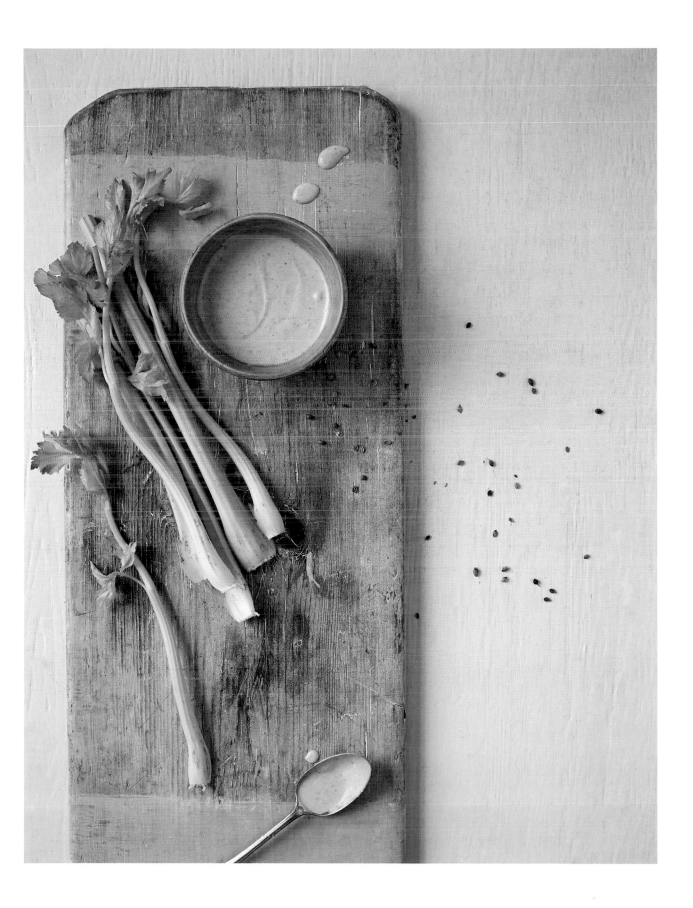

THE GINGERED PEAR

.25 PORTION
PER SERVING

PREP 5 MINS
COOK NIL
SERVES 4

1 ripe pear, peeled and
   cored

2 tbsp olive oil

1 tsp soy sauce

½ tsp balsamic vinegar

½ tsp freshly grated ginger

Place all the ingredients in a blender or food processor and whizz until smooth and creamy. Taste, and tweak the seasoning to your liking, adding more olive oil, vinegar, soy sauce or ginger to suit. Will keep in the fridge for 3–4 days.

Gorgeous with watercress or peppery winter leaves, chicory, thin moons of celery and toasted walnuts.

THE TOMATO

.5 PORTION
PER SERVING

PREP 5 MINS
COOK NIL
SERVES 4

200g fresh tomatoes (any
   colour – yellow makes a
   wickedly sunny dressing)

a pinch of fresh herbs
   (thyme leaves or fresh basil
   work beautifully)

4 tbsp olive oil

sea salt and freshly ground
   black pepper

Place all the ingredients in a blender or food processor and whizz until smooth. Taste, and adjust the seasoning to your liking. Thin out with a little drop of water, if needed. Will keep in the fridge for 3–4 days.

Ideal served with a platter of chopped veg, including cucumber, celery, radishes, lettuce and fennel wedges.

Variation: you can take this dressing in all sorts of directions. Go Mexican with fresh coriander and cumin seeds. Take it to Italy with basil and a drop of balsamic, or travel to Asia with Thai basil and a little lemongrass and ginger. Pick a country, take its key flavours and you've got a whole new creation that'll take your taste buds to exotic lands.

THE ZINGY TAHINI

 PORTION PER SERVING

PREP 10 MINS
COOK NIL
SERVES 4

2 tbsp tahini

1 tbsp olive oil

zest and juice of 1 orange

½ tsp soy sauce

a pinch of chilli powder

Spoon the tahini into a jam jar or bowl. Add the olive oil, orange zest and juice, soy sauce and chilli powder. Give it a swirl with a spoon until well mixed. Trickle in a little water, if needed, to thin it to the desired consistency – you can have it as thick or as thin as you like.

Taste, adding a little more soy sauce or chilli to suit. Will keep in the fridge for a week. Use to drizzle over salads or steamed green beans, or as a dip for just about any veg.

THE GREEK GODDESS HONEY

 PORTION PER SERVING

PREP 10 MINS
COOK NIL
SERVES 4

4 tbsp olive oil

1 tbsp cider, red wine or honey vinegar

1 tbsp water

1 tbsp runny honey

a pinch of ground cinnamon

a sprig of fresh rosemary, leaves finely chopped

½ small garlic clove, finely minced

a pinch of sea salt and freshly ground black pepper

Place all the ingredients in a jam jar. Pop a lid on and give it a good shake. Taste, and tweak the seasoning, if needed. Will keep at room temperature for a couple of days, or in the fridge for 2 weeks.

Perfect for glossing hearty, bitter winter leaves such as chicory, radicchio and mustard greens.

Dips

THE BASICS: Dips are one of the fastest routes to packing in heaps of veg. The following dips offer a portion of veg or two before you've even dunked a carrot stick. Roasting is a great option: aubergines, tomatoes, red peppers, carrots, beetroot, onions, squash, swede . . . the list could go on and on. Pair with a little oil, spice, some nuts or something creamy (yoghurt, mascarpone, cheese) and you're on your way to dipping nirvana.

Raw dips are perfect for the summer. Take a pestle and mortar to the allotment and you'll have the freshest dips in the land. One of my favourite dips of summer is broad bean or pea pesto. Swap the beans for basil or toss both into the mix. Sorrel and mint are also heavenly in the fold.

Then there's houmous, of course. I could probably write an entire cookbook stuffed with variations on the theme, but the basic approach is to make a classic base and then add roast, raw or fried veg and spice. Dried porcini whizzed to a powder is a great addition, or you can swap the chickpeas for easily mashable veg like roast swede. Go for lime instead of lemon and toss in some cumin and thyme leaves for a seriously exciting spread for your pita.

GARDEN GREENS AÏOLI

This recipe looks rather strict and structured, but you can totally play around with the greens here. Swap the basil and mint for tarragon and chive, sorrel and coriander – you name it. Likewise, the watercress can be swapped for more herbs, rocket or your favourite rich green leaf, be it delicate or spicy.

 .5 PORTION PER SERVING (ANY DUNKED VEG IS EXTRA)

PREP 15 MINS
COOK NIL
SERVES 4–6

1 egg yolk

1 tsp Dijon mustard

1 small garlic clove

3 tbsp rapeseed or walnut oil

2 tbsp olive oil

75g watercress

30g fresh basil

30g fresh mint

1 tsp honey (optional)

sea salt and freshly ground black pepper

Pop the egg yolk, mustard, garlic and a pinch of salt and pepper in a blender or food processor and whizz until fully mixed. Keep the motor running as you trickle in the oils, 1 tablespoon at a time, until thick and creamy.

Pack the watercress in and blitz until incorporated. Add the herbs and blitz again until they're fully whipped into the mix and you've got a creamy, relatively thick and frothy dip.

Taste, and whizz in a little honey to soften and round the flavours, if needed, and more salt and pepper, to your liking.

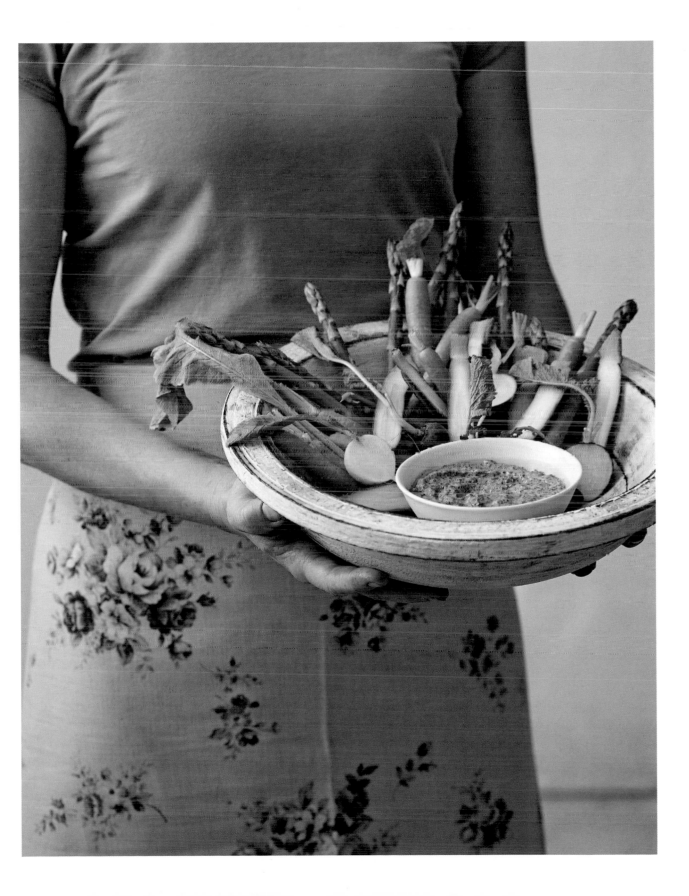

ROAST AUBERGINE, WALNUT AND HARISSA

Sandwiched between a fish and chip shop and a mini cab office is a little door that leads down a long, dimly lit stairwell. Inside exotic lanterns, ornate tea pots, shisha pipes and the smell of warming spices transport you to another land. This is my new local Persian restaurant. On my first visit, I enhaled their amazing, chargrilled walnut and aubergine dip similar to this, but without the harissa, so if you can't get hold of this wonderful spice blend or fancy it without, it's perfectly delicious.

 JUST SHY OF 1 PORTION PER SERVING

PREP   10 MINS
COOK   35 MINS
SERVES   4

1 whole aubergine

a few glosses of olive oil

1 smallish garlic clove

50g walnuts, toasted

½–1 tsp harissa (more or less, to taste)

a little fresh mint, parsley or rosemary, plus extra to garnish

a squeeze of lemon juice (optional)

sea salt and freshly ground black pepper

Preheat the oven to 200°C/Gas 6. Place a roasting tray in the oven to heat up.

Halve the aubergine lengthways. Make 1cm-deep cuts into the flesh of the aubergine at 2–3cm intervals on the diagonal. Repeat in the opposite direction to create a criss-cross pattern. Dust with a hint of salt and a hit of pepper and gloss with a little olive oil. Roast the aubergine on the preheated roasting tray, on a high shelf in the oven for about 35 minutes until tender and bronzed on top.

Pop the roasted aubergine into a blender or food processor (keep the skin on as it lends colour, texture and flavour) with the garlic clove, walnuts, a dab of harissa and your herbs. Whizz until smooth. For a more textured finish, just chop everything together as finely as you can on a large cutting board.

Taste, and add more harissa to suit, dabbing it in little by little. Add a gloss of olive oil and a squeeze of lemon juice, if you like. Finish with a pinch of chopped parsley or a scattering of baby mint leaves.

Wonderful with raw celery, red pepper and toasted triangles of brown sourdough as dippers.

HOMEMADE HARISSA
Chop 50g dried chillies (stems removed) or use chilli flakes. Cover with boiling water and soak for 1 hour. Drain. Place in a food processor with 1 tsp each of fresh mint, ground coriander, ground cumin and honey. Add ¼ tsp ground caraway, 3 peeled garlic cloves and a pinch of salt. Add a pinch of dried rose petals too, if you have them. Whizz for a moment. Scrape down the sides of the bowl, then whizz again, trickling in 50ml of olive oil until its fully mixed. This makes about 300ml which you can store in a sterilised jar in the fridge for up to 6 months.

INDIAN CARROT, CORIANDER AND LIME

When I first made this I asked my 7-year-old son to give it a taste and tell me what he thought. He grabbed a large spoon and ate the lot before I could blink. I gathered it was a goer.

 PORTIONS PER SERVING

PREP 15 MINS (PLUS OVERNIGHT SOAKING IF USING DRIED CHICKPEAS)

COOK 35 MINS

SERVES 4

500g carrots, peeled and cut into 2cm chunks

a gloss of oil (olive, coconut, rapeseed)

1 x 400g tin of chickpeas, drained, or 200g dried chickpeas, soaked overnight and boiled in fresh water until tender

1 garlic clove

1 tsp freshly grated ginger

1 tbsp curry powder

a large handful of fresh coriander or parsley

zest and juice of 2 limes or 1 lemon

3–4 tbsp coconut milk

a pinch of finely chopped fresh red chilli, chilli flakes or chilli powder, to taste

sea salt and freshly ground black pepper

Preheat the oven to 200°C/Gas 6. Place a roasting tray in the oven to heat up.

Toss the carrots in a bowl with a pinch of salt and pepper. Gloss with oil, then tumble into the warmed tin. Roast for 35 minutes, or until fully tender.

Warm the chickpeas in a saucepan for 5 minutes or until warmed through. Drain, then place in a blender or food processor with the garlic, ginger, curry powder, roasted carrots, fresh herbs, and the lime or lemon zest and juice. Whizz, trickling in the coconut milk as you blend, until smooth.

Taste, adding more juice, zest, salt, pepper and chilli to taste. If it's a little too thick or dry, whizz in a little water or oil to reach the desired consistency.

This is striking when served with raw stems of purple sprouting broccoli, but it's absolutely delicious with just about any dippable veg, breadsticks, on toast, in sandwiches and more.

Variation: the combo of roasted carrots, warm chickpeas, curry spices and heaps of fresh coriander is quite beautiful before you go and blend it all up. Indeed, you can easily forgo the dip and turn this into a stunning little salad. Or trickle in some stock and you've got a pretty amazing soup. A swirl of chilli oil on any of these, be it dip, salad or soup, is the perfect finishing touch.

RADISH AND TARRAGON TZATZIKI

 0.5 PORTION PER SERVING (ANY DUNKED VEG IS EXTRA)

PREP **15 MINS**
COOK **NIL**
SERVES **4**

8–10 radishes

1 small garlic clove, finely minced

250g natural or Greek yoghurt

3–4 tbsp finely chopped fresh tarragon leaves●

a drizzle of olive oil

1 lemon

sea salt and freshly ground black pepper

Pluck the tops off the radishes (save them for a salad or turn them into pesto). Scrub the radishes clean, then grate coarsely. Mix with a pinch of salt, pop into a sieve and press out any excess juice.

Add a pinch of salt and pepper and the minced garlic to the yoghurt and mix to combine. Tip the yoghurt into a serving dish and pile the grated radish on top. Scatter over the tarragon leaves.

Drizzle with a little oil, then sprinkle over a grating of lemon zest and a twist of black pepper. Serve layered like this or gently fold everything together ready for dipping.

NOTE: This is best served immediately. If it sits for a while, you may get a little radish liquid weeping out. If so, just drain it off or mix it through again.

● *No tarragon? Swap with fresh mint or dill.*

ARRANQUE ROTENO

This Andalucian dip is similar to gaspacho, making cucumber the perfect dipping accompaniment.

 1 PORTION PER SERVING

PREP **5 MINS**
COOK **NIL**
SERVES **4**

250g ripe tomatoes

75g green pepper●

1 garlic clove

1–2 tbsp breadcrumbs (optional)

a drop of sherry or red wine vinegar

a gloss of olive oil

a handful of fresh parsley, finely chopped, to garnish

sea salt and freshly ground black pepper

Roughly chop the tomatoes and peppers, discarding the stems and the pepper seeds. Scoop out the tomato seeds too if you like (I don't always bother with this).

In a blender or food processor, whizz the veg with the garlic and a hint of salt and pepper. Gradually work in the breadcrumbs until your desired texture is achieved, adding more or less to suit. Taste, and adjust the seasoning, adding a drop of vinegar, to taste.

Finish with a gloss of olive oil and a sprinkling of fresh parsley.

● *Give it a deeper Spanish flavour by swapping the raw green pepper with 100g padron peppers, cooked in a smoking hot frying pan with no oil until lightly charred all over. Remove stems and seeds and blend into the dip.*

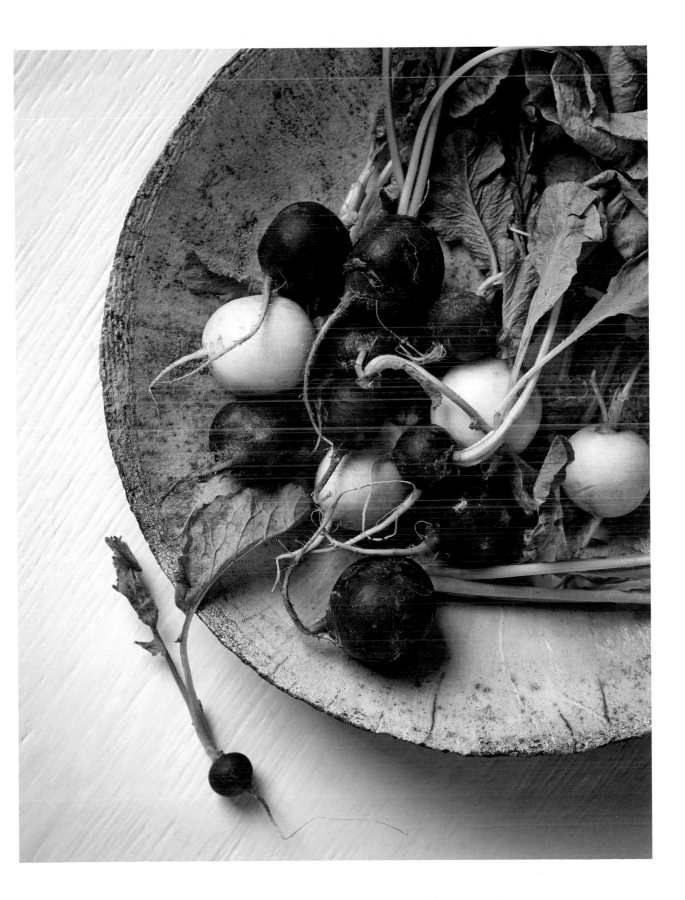

Nibbles

THE BASICS: My friend Joanna is one of the most generous hosts I've ever known. Every time we visit (which is often), she lays on a feast, spinning things effortlessly from her kitchen, like homemade loaves of bread or a tray of roasted squash canapés. I love the idea of something so simple and seasonal being laid out as a party snack. Simply cut some veg into dippable-sized hunks or wedges, then roast until just tender, but still holding its bite and texture. Scatter a little spice, seeds, crushed nuts or herbs over the veg to make it even more inviting, throw in a little dip, then stand back and watch your friends and family fill up on veg.

SESAME AUBERGINE BITES WITH HONEY MISO DIP

 PORTIONS PER SERVING

PREP 10 MINS
COOK 25 MINS
SERVES 4

2 large or 3 medium-sized aubergines

a gloss of olive or rapeseed oil

2 tbsp sesame seeds

sea salt and freshly ground black pepper

FOR THE DRESSING
1 tbsp miso (any kind – I use barley miso)

1 tbsp sesame oil

1 tbsp rice or ½ tsp cider vinegar

2 tbsp water

1 tsp honey

1 small garlic clove, finely minced

a pinch of chilli flakes or finely chopped fresh red chilli

Preheat the oven to 200°C/Gas 6. Place a large roasting tray on the top shelf of the oven to heat up.

Halve the aubergines lengthways and cut each half into hunks (roughly 5 x 3cm). Place in a bowl with a pinch of salt and a good hit of pepper. Gloss with oil and toss to coat. Tumble onto the warmed tray and roast until tender and nicely coloured around the edges, about 25 minutes.

Combine the miso and sesame oil together, slowly whisking in the other ingredients until smooth. Taste, adding a little more water if it's too strong, or additional chilli or garlic if it needs more spice.

Toast the sesame seeds in a dry frying pan until fragrant and just golden. Scatter them over your aubergines as soon as you take them out of the oven, and gently roll them through the seeds to coat.

Pile the aubergine wedges on a plate and serve with the miso dip. Utterly delicious.

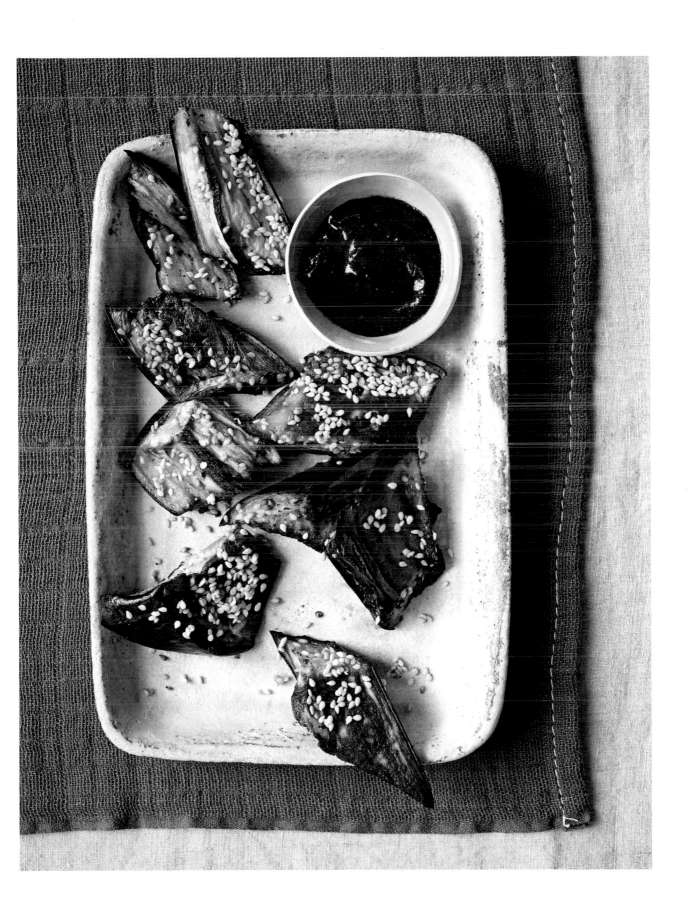

ROAST CUMIN CAULIFLOWER WITH CHIPOTLE LIME CRÈME FRAÎCHE

2 PORTIONS
PER SERVING

PREP 10 MINS
COOK 25 MINS
SERVES 4

½ chipotle or similar
   smoked chilli●

1 head of cauliflower

1 tbsp cumin seeds

2 limes

a gloss of olive or rapeseed
   oil

200g crème fraîche

a handful of fresh coriander
   or parsley leaves (optional)

sea salt and freshly ground
   black pepper

Preheat the oven to 200°C/Gas 6. Place a large roasting tray on the top shelf of the oven to heat up. Soak the chilli in boiling water for 5–10 minutes.

Cut the cauliflower into chunky, dippable-sized hunks (leave a little bit of the stalk on some and any tender leaves attached) and place in a bowl with a little salt and pepper, the cumin seeds, the zest and juice of one of the limes and a gloss of oil. Tumble into the warmed tray and roast until the cauliflower is nicely bronzed around the edges, about 25 minutes.

Drain the soaking chilli, then split it in half and scoop out the seeds and membrane. Chop finely. Wash your hands well afterwards and don't rub your eyes!

Place the crème fraîche in a bowl and add a pinch of salt and pepper along with the zest and a little squeeze of juice from the remaining lime. Add a dot of the chilli, taste, and add more until the heat is just right for you (consider your guests, too – you can always make up a hot dip and a milder one).

Pile the roasted cauli on a serving tray. Scrape any cumin seeds lingering in the pan over the top. Finish with a fresh hit of lime juice and a scattering of fresh coriander or parsley, if liked. Serve alongside the dip.

● *If you can't find a chipotle or smoked chilli, use ½ teaspoon hot smoked paprika, or ½ teaspoon sweet smoked paprika with a pinch of chilli powder, to taste.*

ROAST SQUASH BITES WITH SWEET CHILLI SAUCE

 1 PORTION FOR EVERY
4 HUNKS OF SQUASH

PREP   10 MINS
COOK   30 MINS
SERVES   4

½ a large or 1 smaller squash
   or pumpkin, cut into
   4–5cm chunks •

a gloss of olive oil

a handful of fresh parsley or
   coriander and lime
   wedges, to serve (optional)

sea salt and freshly ground
   black pepper

FOR THE CHILLI SAUCE
75g honey

1 red chilli, finely chopped,
   or 1 tsp chilli flakes (more
   or less, to taste)

1 garlic clove, finely minced

1 tbsp cider vinegar

Preheat the oven to 200°C/Gas 6. Place a large baking or roasting tray in the oven to heat up.

Toss the squash with a little salt and pepper and coat with a gloss of olive oil. Tumble onto the warm baking tray, arranging the pieces in a single layer, and roast in the oven until tender and golden around the edge, about 30 minutes.

Whisk the honey, chilli, garlic and vinegar together for the sauce.

Arrange the roast squash on a cutting board or serving dish. Scatter over the parsley or coriander and serve with the sweet chilli sauce and wedges of lime.

● *If the skin on your squash or pumpkin is thin, leave it on if you like. It's completely edible and adds nice texture.*

ROAST LEMON ASPARAGUS WITH PESTO YOGHURT

1 PORTION
PER SERVING

PREP 10 MINS
COOK 10 MINS
SERVES 4

400g chunky asparagus spears

a gloss of olive or rapeseed oil

1 lemon

200g natural yoghurt

2 tbsp fresh pesto

a scattering of fresh basil leaves (optional)

sea salt and freshly ground black pepper

Preheat the oven to 200°C/Gas 6. Place a large roasting tray on the top shelf of the oven to heat up.

Trim any woody ends off the asparagus. Toss with a little salt, pepper, olive oil, lemon zest and a squeeze of lemon juice. Tumble into the tray and roast for 10 minutes, or until the spears are just tender.

Spoon the yoghurt into a bowl and dollop the pesto in. Make an artful swirl by gently rippling a knife through.

Pile the asparagus on a serving tray alongside the dip. Garnish with fresh basil leaves, if using, curls of lemon zest and a gentle dusting of salt and pepper.

> **PESTO**
> *Pound or blend 1 tbsp toasted pine nuts with 4 tbsp fresh basil leaves, 1 tbsp freshly grated Parmesan and 1 tbsp olive oil until smooth.*

ROAST BEETROOT WITH CARDAMOM YOGHURT

1.5 PORTIONS
PER SERVING

PREP 10 MINS
COOK 45 MINS
SERVES 4

500g beetroot, peeled and cut into 4cm chunks

a small pinch of chilli powder

a gloss of olive oil

200g natural yoghurt

3 cardamom pods, seeds finely ground

a handful of fresh mint leaves

sea salt and freshly ground black pepper

Preheat the oven to 220°C/Gas 7. Place a large roasting tray in the oven to heat up.

Mix the beetroot with a pinch of salt, pepper and chilli powder. Gloss with a little oil and toss to coat. Tumble into the warmed tray and roast until tender and just golden around the edges, about 45 minutes.

Mix the yoghurt with the ground cardamom. Taste, and add a little salt or pepper or cardamom, as needed – or more yoghurt if there's too much cardamom for your taste.

Arrange the beetroot on a serving dish. Season, as needed. Scatter over the fresh mint leaves and serve alongside the yoghurt dip.

> ● *Vegan? Coconut milk yoghurt is a great replacement.*

Toast

THE BASICS: Toast is a great way of turning something light into a meal. Toast mounted with beautiful things is easy to make and looks smashing. While I'm a slave to a good sourdough or a sticky, seedy loaf of rye, you can really have fun by using different breads for your toast. Sweet challah is lovely with ricotta mixed with saffron and honey and topped with banana slices, a drop of lemon juice and chilli flakes. Ciabatta is heavenly with squashed tomatoes, capers and basil.

You can pile any of the slaws or little salads featured in this chapter onto your favourite toast. And the dips, most certainly, make marvellous spreads.

OLIVE RAISIN TAPENADE WITH FENNEL AND ORANGE

 PORTIONS PER SERVING

PREP 15 MINS
COOK NIL
MAKES 4

150g black olives, pitted

75g raisins

2 oranges or 5 clementines

a pinch of chilli flakes or chilli powder (optional)

½ fennel bulb

a few glosses of olive oil

4 pitta breads, toasted

fennel fronds, fresh mint or thyme leaves, to garnish

sea salt and freshly ground black pepper

In a blender or food processor, whizz the olives, raisins and a grating of orange zest to form a rough paste. (No food processor? Just chop the ingredients on a cutting board as finely as you can.) Taste, and add a little chilli, if you like.

Slice the tops and bottoms off the oranges. Stand them on a cutting board and carve the skin off. If using clementines, just peel them. Cut the segments of the oranges/clementines away from their pithy membrane and place them in a bowl, brushing any lingering juice into the bowl with them.

Use a veg peeler to shave the fennel into thin wisps. Drizzle over a little oil and any juice left from cutting the oranges/clementines.

Mound the olive tapenade topping on the toasted pittas, spreading and pressing it across the bread. Top with a layer of fennel wisps, then dot the orange/clementine segments over the top. Gloss with a little oil, and add a hit of salt, pepper and chilli, if you wish. Finish with fennel fronds, mint or thyme leaves.

SPANAKOPITA TOASTIE

1 PORTION PER SERVING

PREP 20 MINS
COOK 15 MINS
SERVES 4

350g spinach

6–8 spring onions, thinly sliced

200g feta, crumbled

1 egg, whisked

a handful of fresh or a pinch of dried dill (optional)

8 slices of sourdough

a gloss of olive oil

freshly ground black pepper

If you've got a toastie machine, warm it up. If not, you can fry these gorgeous Greek-tart-inspired toasties in a frying pan.

In a large bowl, mix the raw spinach with the sliced spring onions, crumbled feta and whisked egg. Add a good pinch of pepper and the dill, if using. Fold everything together until well mixed.

Brush the sides of the bread that will be pressed against the toaster or pan with olive oil. Pile a mound of the cheesy spinach mix in the centre of 4 of the bread slices and cap with the remaining slices.

Carefully transfer to your toastie machine, cooking in batches as needed. Or heat a large frying pan and fry the sandwiches, adding a little extra oil to the pan, if needed, until golden on each side.

Delicious with a big salad of fresh tomatoes mixed with a pinch of salt, olive oil and heaps of fresh herbs.

GRILLED RED PEPPER RIBBONS AND GOAT'S CURD

1 PORTION PER SERVING

PREP 15 MINS
COOK 40 MINS
SERVES 4

2 large or 6 smaller red peppers

4 slices of sourdough or your favourite bread, toasted

a gloss of olive oil

200g goat's curd or Greek yoghurt

a dusting of smoked paprika

3–4 tbsp toasted almonds, crushed or chopped

sea salt and freshly ground black pepper

Preheat the oven to 220°C/Gas 7.

Pop the peppers on a baking tray. Set on the top shelf of the oven and roast for about 30–40 minutes until charred on top and bottom, turning halfway through cooking to achieve this. Once the peppers are ready, remove from the oven and leave to cool.

Gloss the toast slices with a little oil, then slather on the goat's curd or Greek yoghurt. Sprinkle with a little salt and pepper.

When the peppers have cooled, remove the charred skin, stems and seeds. Tear the peppers into ribbons and arrange over the top of the creamy capped toasts. Dust with smoked paprika, dot with the toasted almonds, and finish with a little salt, pepper and a trickle of oil.

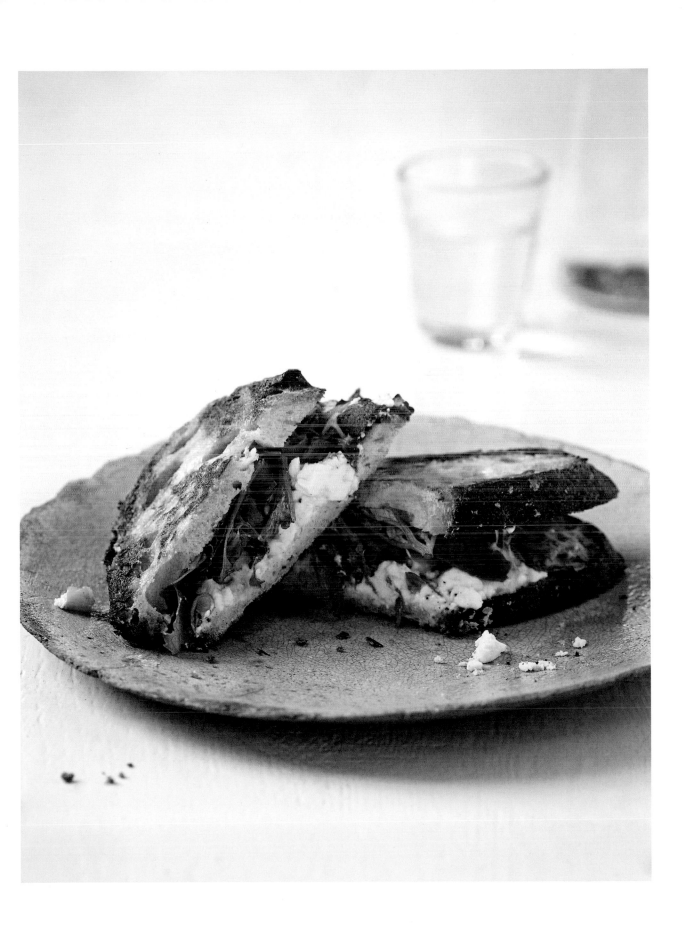

SEEDY AVOCADO TOASTS

 PORTION PER SERVING

PREP 10 MINS
COOK NIL
SERVES 4

4 large or 8 smaller slices of toast

a few glosses of olive oil

2 large or 4 smaller avocados, thinly sliced

2 limes

4 tbsp mixed seeds pumpkin, sunflower, sesame, hemp, linseed), toasted

1 tsp cumin seeds, toasted

a little runny honey

a few chilli flakes (optional)

sea salt

Gloss the toast slices with olive oil and top with the avocado slices. Dust with a pinch of salt and squeeze over a good hit of lime juice.

Scatter the toasted seeds over the top and finish with a little honey, an extra pinch of salt and a hint of chilli, if you like.

Delicious with the Black Bean and Smoked Pepper Soup on page 57.

PEAS ON TOAST WITH CHORIZO

 PORTIONS PER SERVING

PREP 10 MINS
COOK NIL (OR 10 MINS IF COOKING CHORIZO)
SERVES 4

500g frozen peas

1 smallish garlic clove

1 lemon or lime

1–2 tsp olive oil

100g cured or cooking chorizo

4 large or 8 smaller slices of toast (sourdough works a treat here)

sea salt and freshly ground black pepper

Rinse the peas under warm water until tender, then place in a blender or food processor with the garlic, a pinch of salt and pepper, a squeeze of lemon or lime juice and a teaspoon of olive oil. It won't be silky smooth unless you pass it through a sieve, but then you lose all the texture and healthy fibrous bits. The key is to get it smooth enough to spread and hold on the toast, which simply crushing the peas doesn't quite achieve. Trickle in a little more olive oil or lemon/lime juice if needed and adjust the seasoning, to taste.

If using cured chorizo, thinly slice if it's not sliced already. For cooking chorizo, get a frying pan hot. Squeeze the chorizo meat out of its skin. Crumble into the hot pan. Fry for 5–10 minutes, until just golden and cooked through. Set aside.

Gloss the toast with a little oil. Spoon and smooth the peas over and top with the chorizo.

Variation: replace the chorizo with shreds of leftover roast lamb, crumbled nuggets of feta, fried slices of salty halloumi or simply curls of lemon zest, salted black olives and fresh mint.

Slaws

THE BASICS: Forget the soggy veg, mayo-drenched stuff you buy in the supermarket. Get out your box grater. Eating coleslaw will become a whole new experience. Throw in a little fruit and you pretty much eradicate the need for a dressing. Fruit takes care of the zingy acidic kick and sweet foil offered by a good dressing. It also sneaks in more vitamins and lends a great textural contrast. And as with most things, spices, nuts and seeds are like the icing on the cake.

A box grater or a food processor with a grating attachment helps you get the job done, but you could always julienne your fruit and veg (cut it into little matchsticks) for a more textured effect. It takes longer but makes for a richer-looking plate of food.

COCONUT CRAB AND KALE CORONATION

2 PORTIONS
PER SERVING

PREP 10 MINS
COOK 5 MINS
SERVES 4

200g kale or cavolo nero

200ml coconut milk

1 tbsp curry powder

200g crab meat (a mix of brown and white is perfect, but either one on their own is fine)

1 lime

4 tbsp desiccated coconut or coconut flakes, toasted

sea salt and freshly ground black pepper

Tug the kale leaves from their woody stalks (you can finely slice the stalks and toss them into the mix, or add them to a juice mix). Stack the leaves on top of each other (you can do this in batches), roll up and thinly slice, giving you near-paper-thin ribbons.

If you're not a hard-core raw green eater (I'm possibly alone when it comes to my love of munching on raw kale), tumble the kale ribbons into a fine mesh sieve and pour boiling water over the kale to soften the leaves a little. Shake dry. Or go for the raw kale if you fancy.

Whisk the coconut milk and curry powder together in a large serving bowl. Pile the kale and crab meat on top. Grate in some lime zest. Squeeze in a good hit of lime juice. Fold everything together. Taste. Add more curry powder, coconut milk and/or a little salt and pepper, if needed. Finish with a scattering of the toasted coconut.

ELLA'S HAITIAN LIME AND CHILLI WITH BANANA PEZÉE

Most Saturdays I help run a local food stall at Crystal Palace Food Market. Early February is a pretty lean month for local food, but on one occasion we were surprised by the arrival of the most enormous cabbage I'd ever seen. Sharing in my admiration for this bountiful brassica, Ella Wright, who was on the stall with me, shared this corker of a recipe, which she picked up in French Guiana.

 2.5 PORTIONS
PER SERVING

PREP 10 MINS
COOK NIL
SERVES 4

1 large carrot, grated

1 small onion or 2 shallots, chopped

½ large cabbage, finely chopped

1 chilli (Ella suggests Scotch Bonnet) (more or less, to taste)

1 veg stock cube, crushed●

zest and juice of 1 lime

a handful of fresh coriander or parsley, chopped (optional)

Mix the carrot, onion and cabbage in a large bowl.

Remove the seeds and membrane from the chilli, and chop finely. Pop in a bowl with the crushed stock cube and mix together. Add the lime zest and juice and mix again.

Fold into the vegetables and finish with the fresh herbs. Serve with Banane Pezée.

● *No stock cube? Use 1½ tsp of curry powder (more or less, to taste) instead. If your curry powder is on the spicy side, use less chilli or skip it altogether.*

BANANA PEZÉE
To make banana pezée, peel 4 plantain and cut each into 5 pieces. Soak in salted water for 10 minutes, then drain and pat dry. Heat a gloss of sunflower oil in a frying pan then shallow fry the plantain over a medium heat until just starting to colour. Remove from pan and squish the pieces between 2 saucers until they're ½–1cm flat. Return the squished fritters to the frying pan and sizzle until golden and crispy. Finish with a squeeze of lime.

APPLE AND PARMESAN WITH WALNUTS AND WATERCRESS

This recipe started as an apple, walnut and blue cheese pesto. My colleague Paul Freestone made it for Abel & Cole's daily lunch club one day when I wasn't in. The emails that were flying around praising it were torture, but I made a note of the idea and have held on to it since. When I opened my fridge to make it, I realised I was out of blue cheese so I tried Parmesan instead and fell in love with this recipe. It's the sort of thing you can rustle up in minutes when you need a quick hunger fix.

 1.5 PORTIONS PER SERVING

PREP   5 MINS
COOK   NIL
SERVES   4

80g walnuts, toasted and chopped

4 apples, coarsely grated

50g Parmesan, finely grated

100g watercress (or rocket)

a drop of olive or walnut oil

1 lemon

a pinch of black pepper

Combine the walnuts, apples and Parmesan in a bowl. Toss with the watercress. Gloss with a little oil and add a little grated lemon zest and juice. Taste. Season and tweak ingredient balance to your liking.

Variation: for the pesto option, whizz the walnuts, apples and Parmesan with a heap of parsley or watercress (about 50g), trickling in enough walnut or olive oil to bring it all together. Season to taste.

FENNEL AND PINEAPPLE WITH AVOCADO AND CHILLI CASHEWS

 1.5 PORTIONS PER SERVING

PREP 15 MINS
COOK NIL
SERVES 4

1 large or 2 small fennel bulb(s)

¼ large or ½ small pineapple

2 ripe avocados

a gloss of olive oil

1 tsp fennel seeds, toasted

a pinch of chilli flakes

a handful of cashews, toasted

a handful of fresh coriander or mint leaves (optional)

sea salt and freshly ground black pepper

Quarter the fennel bulb. Use a veg peeler or mandolin to cut into thin, wispy slivers.

Peel the pineapple but keep it in 1 or 2 large chunks. Grate it over the fennel. The pineapple will not grate into perfect shreds but becomes more like a thick purée/dressing for the fennel; this works a treat, making it extra juicy and lush.

Halve your avocados. Pop the stones out. Remove the peel. Cut into thin moons.

Mix a pinch of salt and pepper in with your fennel and pineapple Arrange the mix into bowls or a large serving platter. Tuck the avocado slices into the mix.

Gloss the salad with a little olive oil. Sprinkle the toasted fennel seeds and chilli flakes over. Finish with the toasted cashews and fresh coriander, mint and/or any fennel fronds. Taste. Add more seasoning, if needed.

A stunning side dish for pan-fried bream or grilled squid.

BEETROOT, ORANGE AND POPPY

 1.5 PORTIONS PER SERVING

PREP 15 MINS
COOK NIL
SERVES 4

500g beetroot, peeled and coarsely grated

a tiny pinch of chilli powder

zest and juice of 2 oranges

a few glosses of olive oil

1 tbsp poppy seeds, lightly toasted

sea salt and freshly ground black pepper

Mix the beetroot with a little salt, pepper and chilli powder.

Sprinkle over the orange zest (saving a little to add at the end), so you can see the colour contrast. Squeeze over a good hit of fresh orange juice; taste as you add it and stop when the beetroot is sweet and nicely juicy, but not oversaturated.

Add a gloss of olive oil and half the poppy seeds and mix through. Finish with an extra drizzle of oil, a pinch of sea salt, a final grating of zest and the remaining poppy seeds.

Delicious with roast lamb or grilled mackerel, or bundled into a wrap with fried slices of halloumi and fresh mint.

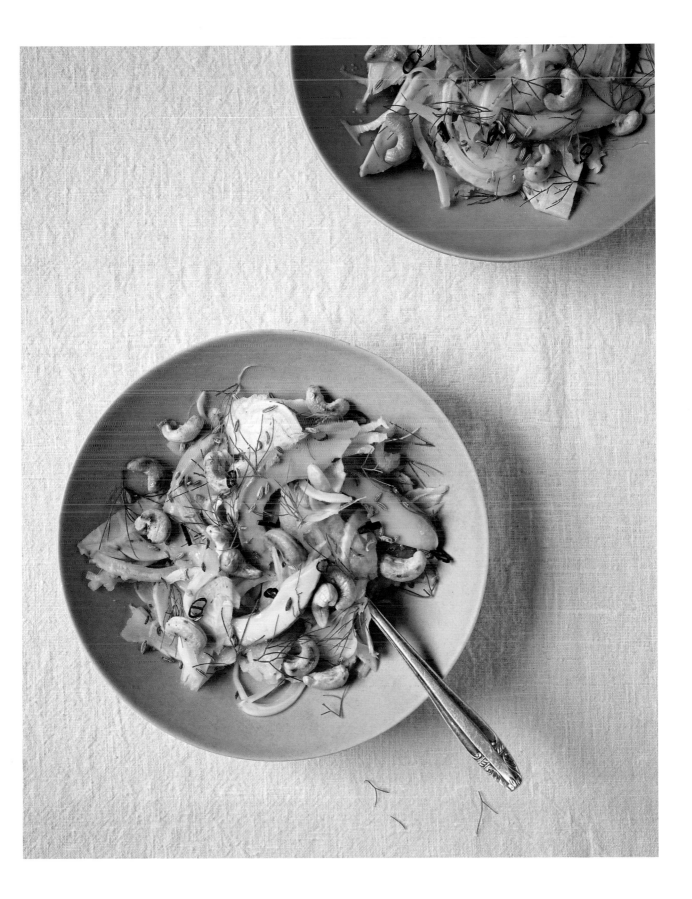

Latkes

THE BASICS: There are as many names for these grated veg fritters as there are flavour possibilities. I must have tried out about 20 variations before deciding on the recipes below.

It was difficult settling on the name. While you could arguably say they're rostis, latke is the Jewish name for these little pancakes. In Sweden they call them rårakor or raggmunk (depending on whether or not you use egg, dairy and flour in the mix), but that's even harder to pronounce, and the recipes below show how these little pancakes can be made with or without eggs and dairy. I find the flour is essential, however. It prevents them from sticking, but again you can be crafty, using anything from garam to rye flour.

These are a brilliant one-man snack, so if you're hungry and don't want to feed a crowd, make yourself a batch of latkes with the bits and bobs you have in your fridge, using the following recipes as a guide.

CARROT, FETA AND DILL

 1 PORTION FOR EVERY 4 LATKES

PREP 15 MINS
COOK 15 MINS
MAKES 16

320g carrots, coarsely grated

1 garlic clove, finely minced

150g feta cheese, crumbled

a good pinch of freshly ground black pepper

a handful of fresh dill leaves, chopped

2 eggs, beaten

50g flour (plain white, gluten-free, kamut)

a little oil, for frying

In a large bowl, mix the grated carrots with the garlic, crumbled feta, freshly ground pepper and dill.

Fold in the eggs, ensuring they're evenly distributed, then dust the flour over and gently fold through.

Heat a large frying pan and gloss with enough oil to lightly coat the pan.

Gather the mix into golf ball-sized mounds and gently dollop each mound into the pan in a single layer (test one first and adjust the eggs/flour ratio accordingly if it sticks or is too wet). Press to flatten. Cook in batches until golden and crisp on each side, adding more oil as needed.

Delicious warm with a dollop of cold Greek yoghurt and fresh dill on top, or pair with a sweet and spicy chilli jam. I love these for brunch.

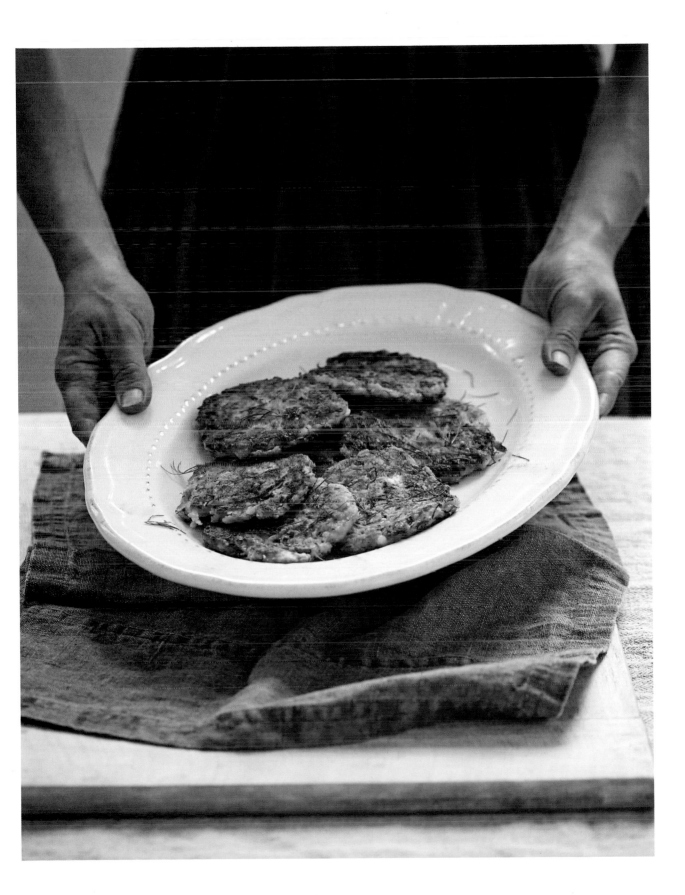

CELERIAC, PEAR AND HAZELNUT WITH GOAT'S CURD

 PORTION FOR EVERY 4 LATKES

PREP 15 MINS
COOK 15 MINS
MAKES 16

250g peeled celeriac, coarsely grated

100g pear, coarsely grated

50g hazelnuts, finely chopped and toasted

1 garlic clove, chopped

a pinch of chopped rosemary

150g goat's curd or similar soft, crumbly, mild cheese

2 eggs, beaten

4 tbsp flour (any variety)

a gloss of oil

sea salt and freshly ground black pepper

In a large bowl, mix the celeriac, pear, nuts, garlic, herbs, salt and pepper until all the ingredients are evenly distributed.

Fold in the cheese, mushing it into the mix. If the mix is quite sticky and can easily form a ball, you may not need the egg (it's there to act as a glue, but sometimes your pear and cheese combined will do this job). Add the eggs only if needed.

The texture of pears varies enormously so if your mix is too wet, sprinkle in a little flour, a tablespoon at a time, until the mix looks manageable.

Heat a large frying pan and add a gloss of oil or ghee. Add a rounded tablespoon of the mix to the pan. Press it flat with the back of a spatula and cook until golden on both sides. Before adding several to the pan, I like to cook one as a tester and then adjust the flour/egg ratio accordingly.

Delicious warm alongside a mound of watercress with fresh pear slices, a trickle of olive oil, a hit of lemon zest and juice and a pinch of salt.

JAPANESE CABBAGE, GINGER AND SESAME

 PORTION FOR EVERY 4 LATKES

PREP 15 MINS
COOK 20 MINS
MAKES 16

200g green cabbage

75g spring onion or leek

50g carrot, coarsely grated

1 tbsp toasted sesame seeds

1 tbsp soy sauce

1 tbsp freshly grated ginger

2 eggs, beaten

4 tbsp plain flour

a gloss of oil

Finely shred the cabbage and thinly slice the spring onion or leek. Mix together the cabbage, spring onions or leeks, grated carrot, sesame seeds, soy sauce and ginger.

Add the egg and scrunch it into the mix using your hands. Dust the flour over and gently mix through.

Heat a large frying pan and add a gloss of oil. Gather the mix into golf ball-sized mounds and gently dollop each mound into the pan in a single layer (test one first and adjust the flour/egg ratio accordingly). Press to flatten. Cook in batches until golden and crisp on each side, adding more oil as needed.

Delicious on their own, hot from the pan. Or add a generous dash of Sriracha, soy or hoisin sauce.

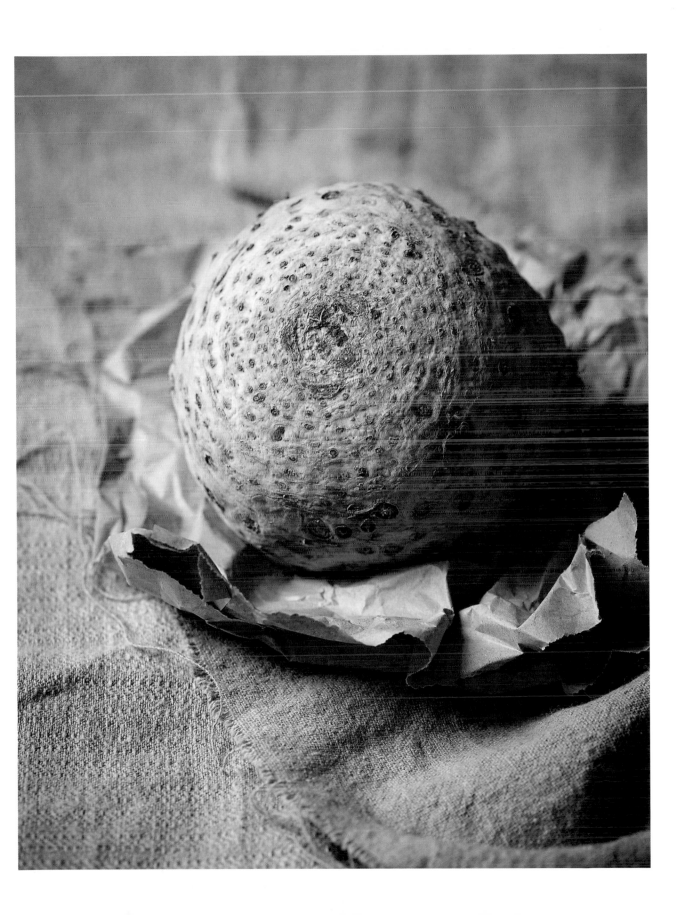

SWEDE AND CHEDDAR

PORTION FOR EVERY 4 LATKES

PREP 15 MINS
COOK 15 MINS
MAKES 16

350g swede, coarsely grated

150g Cheddar or similar cheese, coarsely grated

1 tbsp cumin seeds, toasted

a handful of chopped coriander or thyme leaves

a pinch of smoked paprika or chilli powder

2 eggs, beaten

4 tbsp plain white flour or cornmeal

a little olive or rapeseed oil

Mix the swede, Cheddar, cumin, and herbs and paprika or chilli in a bowl.

Pour in the egg and mix well. Dust the flour, polenta or cornmeal over the top and gently fold through. If the mix is looking a little wet, dust in a little more flour, polenta or cornmeal. You want the mixture moist but not wet-looking.

Heat a large frying pan and gloss with enough oil to lightly coat the pan.

Gather the mix into golf ball-sized mounds and gently dollop each mound into the pan in a single layer (test one first and adjust the polenta/egg ratio accordingly). Press to flatten. Cook in batches until golden and crisp on each side, adding more oil as needed.

Lovely on their own or delicious with a splash of hot chilli sauce or paired with avocado slices and smoked or oven-roast tomatoes.

COURGETTE AND COCONUT

PORTION FOR EVERY 4 LATKES

PREP 15 MINS
COOK 15 MINS
MAKES 16

350g courgettes, coarsely grated

150g desiccated coconut

a pinch of sea salt

1 red chilli, finely chopped

2 tsp cumin seeds

a large handful of chopped fresh coriander and/or mint

4 tbsp coconut milk

50g flour (any variety)

a little oil

Squeeze the excess water out of the courgettes, then mix the courgette with the coconut, a pinch of sea salt, chilli, cumin and herbs.

Fold in the coconut milk, then dust the flour over and gently fold through.

Heat a large frying pan and gloss with enough oil to lightly coat the pan.

Gather the mix into golf ball-sized mounds and gently dollop each mound into the pan in a single layer (test one first and adjust the flour/milk ratio accordingly). Press to flatten. Cook in batches until golden and crisp on each side, adding more oil as needed.

Lovely spritzed with lime juice and eaten warm. Also delicious served with raita (minty yoghurt) or plain natural or Greek yoghurt, or mango chutney for a vegan option.

Liquid lunch

THE BASICS: Juices are one of the best ways to pump a bundle of energy and health-giving vitamins into your body. They're also great to serve to guests: offer them up as a virgin or fully leaded cocktail (just add a shot of your favourite tipple – gin is lovely with Rosy Cheeks). Juices are also great to take to work to stave off sweet cravings or as a healthy liquid lunch.

My favourite piece of kitchen kit is my Samson juicer. I've had it for more than a decade and bought it on the recommendation of Daphne Lambert, a nutritionist and medicinal chef, who runs an organic cookery school, Greencuisine, on the Welsh Borders. She suggested an 'auger' style juicing machine, as the slow rotational squeezing preserves enzymes for healthier juice. (It's also brilliant in that it can make fruit ice creams, nut butters, milks and so much more.) If you don't have a juicer, see the Fruit Shakes in the Breakfast chapter, or give the Salsa Crush or Kale Colada a whirl in a food processor. Whizz the ingredients until they look soupy, then press through a sieve, removing all the pulpy bits.

Speaking of pulpy bits, I hate wasting these energy-rich scraps. I have a few window boxes and I always keep one dormant, full of spent compost, to which I add my juice pulp and veg stock scraps. In a couple of weeks, it's ready to plant in.

You can juice any fruit or veg, and I get a lot of inspiration from simply seeing what's in my fridge or garden. But I also trawl the web looking at the menus of LA juice joints as they seem to be first when it comes to winning juice and smoothie combos. A few veg worth adding to your juice blends: pumpkin (lovely with apple, then shaken with vanilla), celeriac (gorgeous with pear), and fennel (outrageously refreshing with pineapple, cucumber and mint).

Spices and herbs are great to add to juices to keep them interesting. Shake them up with the juice once it's made, or feed them in with the fruit and your juicer will crush some of their oils out (though don't plunge a whole cinnamon stick into your juicer). Likewise, be mindful of seeds: I destroyed my juicer while trying to juice 3kg of foraged blackberries.

The quantity of fruit and veg needed for each juice varies hugely, however as a rough guide, juicing 250g of fruit or veg should give you around 150ml of juice.

CARROT BLOSSOM

 1 PORTION PER SERVING

PREP 10 MINS
COOK NIL
SERVES 1

300g carrots
½ tsp orange blossom water

Scrub the carrots clean and roughly chop. Feed through your juicer, then swirl the orange blossom water in. If you're not drinking it straightaway, shake before serving.

This is a beautiful juice to serve with the Persian Feast on page 171. The vibrant colour and flavour sets the tone wonderfully.

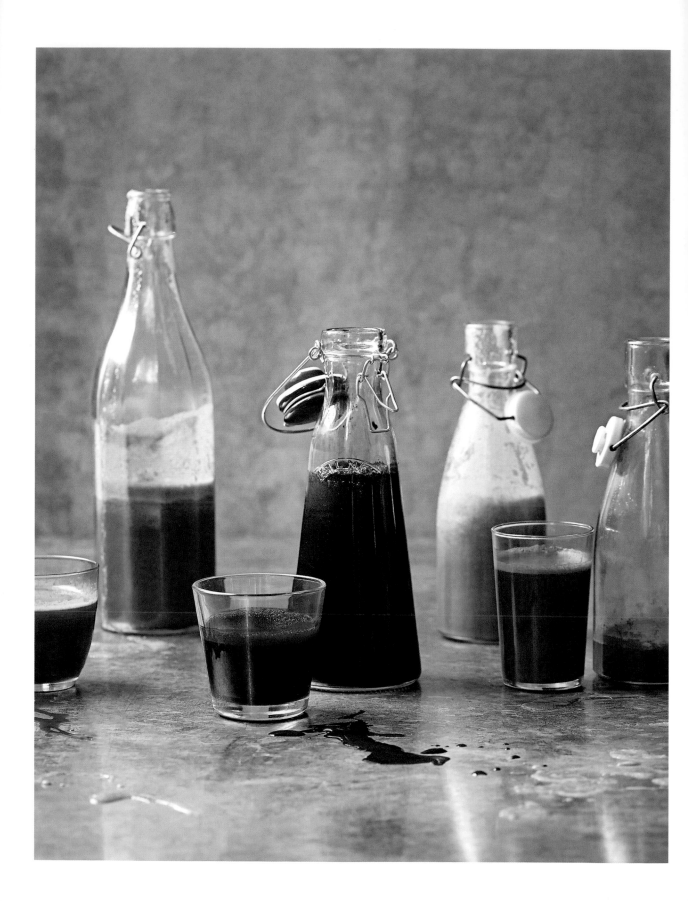

ROSY CHEEKS

Marry the tanginess of rhubarb with the rich, earthy sweetness of beetroot, rounded off with their favourite spice and you've got an absolutely beautiful juice. This has become one of my favourite juices and it's a great way of putting two quintessentially English veg to good use.

 1 PORTION
PER SERVING

PREP 10 MINS
COOK NIL
SERVES 1

100g rhubarb
20g beetroot
1cm slice of fresh ginger

Scrub the rhubarb and beetroot clean. You don't have to peel the beetroot, but if the skin's gone wrinkly or is caked with earth, then it might be wise to. Chop the veg into hunks and feed into the juicer with the ginger. Take a sip, and add a little more ginger, if you like, but don't add too much or it'll overpower the other ingredients.

SOUR APPLE

Sorrel is one of my absolute favourite things to grow and eat. The spinach-like leaves have the most incredible lemony tang, and funnily enough, children seem to go wild for the stuff.

 1 PORTION
PER SERVING

PREP 10 MINS
COOK NIL
SERVES 1

200g apples
50g sorrel●
a splash of cold water

Wash the fruit and leaves. Roughly chop the apples (don't worry about peeling them) and leaves and feed through your juicer. I like to take the edge off this one (and any apple-based juices), by adding a splash of cold water to it before serving. It rounds the flavours off nicely.

> ● *If you can't get hold of sorrel, swap it with any green leaf: spinach, kale, cavolo nero, watercress. Add a squeeze of lemon juice at the end to bring forth that sorrel-like tang, which is the perfect foil to the apple's sweetness and the richness of the greens.*

TROPICAL KALE

Inspired by an LA juice café, where they make a Greeña Colada, this juice takes a similar route of pairing hearty, good-for-you greens with the sweet tropical vibes of pineapple.

 1 PORTION
PER SERVING

PREP 10 MINS
COOK NIL
SERVES 1

50g kale
250g pineapple flesh

Wash the greens, then roughly chop the pineapple and kale. Feed through your juicer along with the mint. Taste, and adjust the balance of ingredients if you like.

Variation: transform the juice into a smoothie by blending this mix with ½ an avocado, 100ml coconut water or 50ml coconut milk, 50ml water and a squeeze of fresh lime juice.

SALSA CRUSH: TOMATO, RED PEPPER, CHILLI AND GARLIC

My Abel & Cole colleague Paul Freestone came up with this juice when we were road testing ideas for the veg box scheme's own juice range, which is made with outgrade fruit and veg (all the ugly, unloved veg that is not quite good enough for the supermarkets). It makes a wicked base for a Bloody Mary.

 1 PORTION
PER SERVING

PREP 10 MINS
COOK NIL
SERVES 1

200g ripe tomatoes
1 red pepper
a slice of red chilli (more or less, to taste)
1 small garlic clove (optional)
2–3 sprigs fresh coriander
a squeeze of lime juice

Roughly chop the tomatoes and pepper, discarding the pepper's seeds and stalk. Feed through your juicer, adding the chilli a thin slice at a time. Taste after each addition to check the heat. Press the garlic and coriander through the juicer and finish with a squeeze of lime juice.

BITE: WILD THINGS

I learned to gather from the experts. Now I find it impossible to go anywhere without seeing free food opportunities. Foraging is incredibly primitive. It connects you with nature by making you look at plants in a whole new light: a source of sustenance.

Dandelions: Bright, sunshiny yellow flowers in spring, with bitter and peppery, rocket-like leaves at the base. Gather some of these from a private garden or another dog-free zone and scatter both leaves and flowers (pluck the yellow petals from their base) into the *Souk Salad* on page 106.

Nettles: These iron-rich leaves look like mint. They grow to about a metre tall and have tiny little hairs on the leaves and stalks. If you pick with gloves and scissors, you'll save yourself a sting. Once cooked, they taste like spinach and totally lose their sting. Gather a bundle for the *Wild Spring Spaghetti* on page 120.

Wild garlic: The leaves of wild garlic look a bit like tulip leaves – wide and smooth. But break one in half: if it smells like garlic, it is indeed wild garlic. It likes the shade and grows best in woodland. The best time to find it is early spring. As well as the *Wild Spring Spaghetti*, you can feature wild garlic in the *Wild Mushrooms Hot Pot* on page 161.

Fennel seeds: If you know the smell and taste of fennel, and are familiar with its green fronds, it's unmistakably easy to find. I think it was the first thing I felt comfortable foraging. The seeds are formed and ready to gather early in the autumn, around September. In summer, the future seed heads will be full of yellow flowers. If you don't know where to gather some near you, it's easy to grow your own. Bronze fennel's my favourite. They're delicious in the *Chard Dolmades* on page 110.

Rosehips: These are the fruits that form once all the petals from wild or cultivated rose in your garden have fallen. The rosehips I know and love tend to come from wild Dogrose shrubs that form part of a native English hedgerow, but I've also cooked with rosehips from garden rose bushes with equal success. My favourite use for them is to make a delicious tea (see page 17), or you can take the pulp used to make the tea, sweeten it further and use it as a syrup over ice cream or fruit, like poached pears or apples. It's beautiful drizzled over warm apple pie.

Other wild things I love: *Ground elder, Jack by the Hedge, wild cabbage, yarrow, Oxeye daisy flowers and leaves, elderflowers, elderberries, bay leaves, and the wild versions of fruits we all know and love: apples, pears and plums. In the autumn, if you spy any of these fruits on a pavement or ground near you, look up. It's likely a fruit-laden tree is hanging above you.*

FAST

Big Salads

THE BASICS: I'd define a salad as a medley of vegetables bound with a dressing of sorts. That's the canvas. From there you can go crazy. Texture is key. Get some crunchy bits in there (croutons, toasted nuts, crispy fried noodles or onions) and marry them with soft, delicate leaves or herbs. A good dressing is what makes the whole thing irresistible.

Making a meal out of a salad is almost like turning a dish inside out. The idea is to let the meat or carbs take the backseat while the veg steps to the fore.

LAZY INDIAN SUMMER SALAD

4 PORTIONS
PER SERVING

PREP   10 MINS (LONGER IF
           USING DRIED CHICKPEAS)
COOK 15 MINS
SERVES 4

2 tbsp curry powder

200g natural, Greek or
coconut milk yoghurt

2 carrots

1 cucumber

2 limes or 1 lemon

a large handful of fresh
mint and/or coriander
leaves

a few glosses of oil (olive,
rapeseed, coconut, ghee)

2 onions, thinly sliced

800g tinned chickpeas,
drained

4 baby gem, cos or similar
crisp lettuces (not
iceberg)

6 tbsp cashews, toasted

sea salt and freshly ground
black pepper

Swirl 2 teaspoons of curry powder into the yoghurt. Taste, and add a pinch of salt and/or more curry powder, if needed.

Cut the carrots and cucumber into ribbons using your veg peeler. Once you get to the seedy core of the cucumber, thinly slice it. Toss the veg into a bowl with a pinch of salt and pepper. Grate in the zest of 1 lime or ½ a lemon along with a good squeeze of juice. Toss in half the herbs. Arrange the salad on individual plates or a large serving platter.

Heat a large frying pan and add a gloss of oil. Tumble the onions into the pan and sizzle over a medium heat until golden and tender. Add the chickpeas, the remaining curry powder and the zest and juice of 1 lime or ½ a lemon. Cook until the chickpeas sizzle and pop, and everything is warmed through. Taste, season as needed, and add more curry powder or citrus to suit.

Scatter the onions and the chickpeas over the carrot and the cucumber ribbons.

Halve the baby gems or if using a larger crisp lettuce, quarter it, keeping the base that holds it together intact.

Add a little more oil to the pan. Place the lettuces in, cut side down, and cook over a medium heat until nicely charred. This only takes a minute. Perch the charred lettuces on top of the salad, then gently fold them into the mix. Scatter the toasted cashews and the remaining herbs over the salad. Serve the curried yoghurt alongside to dollop on the salad as you eat it.

● *If you don't have a cookable lettuce or don't fancy the idea, just skip this bit and use a couple of handfuls of your favourite salad leaves.*

BIG FAT GREEK SALAD WITH JASSY'S FRIED FETA

Jassy Davis is a genius food writer, blogger, author and now a colleague of mine. Of the many wonderful dishes of hers I've tried, her fried feta is one of my favourites – simple, quick and utterly delicious. It's certainly the icing on this wonderfully healthy salad.

 5 PORTIONS
PER SERVING

PREP   15 MINS
COOK   10 MINS
SERVES 4

1 red onion, thinly sliced

1kg tomatoes (try a mix of colours if available)

1 tsp fresh oregano or thyme leaves

2 tbsp red wine vinegar

a little olive oil

1 cucumber, thinly sliced

2 peppers (a mix of colours), cut into rounds (seeds and stem discarded)

4 tbsp pitted olives or 2 tbsp capers (or a combo)

300–400g feta

2 tbsp plain white flour (gluten-free flour also works)

a gloss of runny honey

zest of 1 lemon

a large handful of fresh herbs (dill, mint, basil, parsley, coriander, chervil, chives)

sea salt and freshly ground black pepper

Place the thinly sliced onions in a bowl and pour boiling water over them. Leave to soak and soften while you make up the rest of the salad.

Slice the tomatoes (or halve if they're cherry tomatoes). Sprinkle with the oregano or thyme and a pinch of salt and pepper. Splash the vinegar over. Arrange on your plates or a serving platter and add a drizzle of olive oil.

Scatter the cucumber and pepper slices over the top. Drain the onions and add them to the salad along with the mixed leaves. Gently fold through the tomatoes and dot the olives and/or capers on top.

Cut the feta into 4 large chunks. Soak the cheese in water for a minute, then dust with the flour, coating well on all sides. Heat a large frying pan and add a gloss of oil. Add the feta and fry until golden on all sides.

Top the salad with the feta. Add a very faint gloss of honey and follow with a drizzle of olive oil. Dust with a pinch of salt and pepper and scatter over the lemon zest. Finish with the herbs.

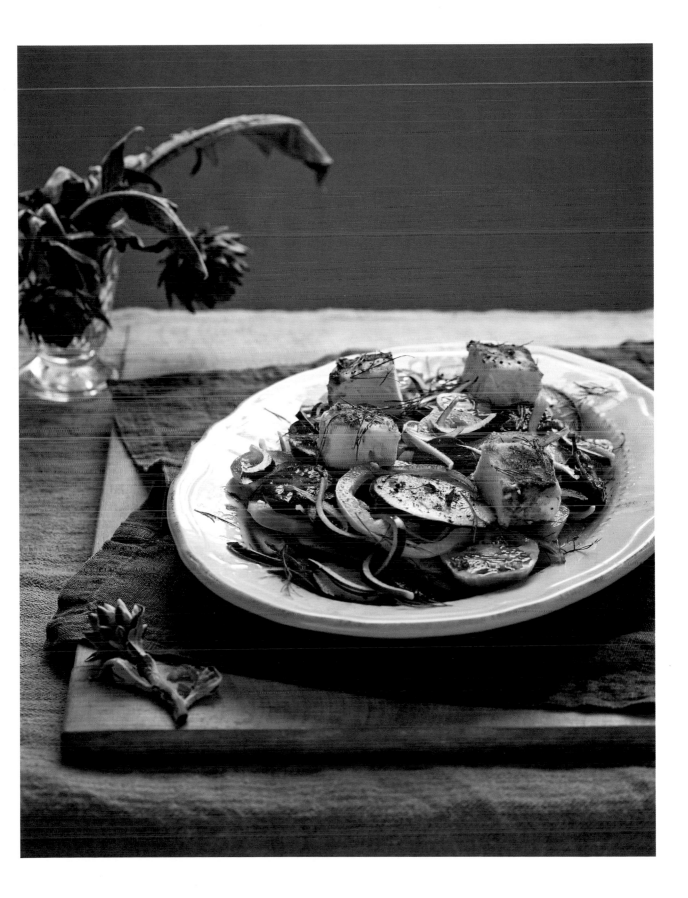

SPANISH BUTTER BEAN TAPAS

This salad is the marriage of two really amazing meals. The first was a beautiful lunch laid on by my Catalan friend, Demi. The lunch featured all the Spanish classics: piquillo peppers, creamy white beans, griddled asparagus, Marcona almonds, gorgeous sausages, sweet, herby Spanish olive oil, smoked paprika.

Not long after that sumptuous feast, I had lunch in La Fromagerie, a gorgeous little London cheese shop with an outstanding café. I had an unforgettable yet simple salad involving a butter bean purée topped with delicate spring veg: raw crunchy peas, radishes and a smattering of fresh herbs.

This dish makes a beautiful supper, or you can serve it as a party platter along with a basket of warm bread.

④ PORTIONS PER SERVING

PREP   20 MINS
COOK   15 MINS
SERVES 4

800g butter beans from a tin or a jar, or 200g dried butter beans soaked overnight and cooked until tender

1 garlic clove, finely minced

zest and juice of 2 lemons

1–2 tbsp olive oil, plus extra for drizzling

a pinch of smoked paprika, plus extra to finish

1 sprig of fresh rosemary, leaves finely chopped

12–16 asparagus spears •

8–12 spring onions •

8 piquillo peppers • •

100g cured chorizo, thinly sliced (optional)

2 tbsp capers (optional)

a good handful of fresh rocket or peppery leaves

sea salt and freshly ground black pepper

Warm the butter beans in a pan in the juices from the tin, or in the cooking liquid if you've cooked them from dried. Drain once steamy and tender, 5–10 minutes. Place in a blender or food processor with the garlic, lemon zest and juice, olive oil, a pinch of paprika, rosemary and salt and pepper. Whizz until smooth, then taste and adjust the seasoning as needed. Set aside and keep covered and warm.

Heat a large frying or griddle pan until smoking hot. Trim the asparagus and spring onions, then rinse, allowing a little water to cling to them. Add to the hot pan (you don't need oil). Cook for a few minutes on each side until just tender and lightly charred. If you have any lemon juice left, squeeze a little over. Season with salt and pepper.

Paint your butter bean purée onto plates using the back of a spoon, creating a bed for the other ingredients to lay upon. Drape the griddled veg over, then tear the red peppers into ribbons and dot them around the plate, along with the chorizo and capers, if using. Artfully scatter the rocket over (this dish is like creating an edible painting) and finish with a drizzle of olive oil and a dusting of smoked paprika.

• *Swap the asparagus and spring onions for any beautiful seasonal veg that grabs you. Slices of fresh summer tomatoes and griddled Padrón peppers are gorgeous. In autumn, opt for roasted shallots and pumpkin wedges.*

• • *No jarred peppers? Roast 2 large red peppers or 4 ramiro peppers on the top shelf of an oven preheated to 200°C/Gas 6, turning once, until nicely charred all over, about 30 minutes.*

BAJA BEACH SALAD WITH CITRUS CHICKEN SKEWERS

 3 PORTIONS
PER SERVING

PREP 15 MINS
COOK 25 MINS
SERVES 4

500g chicken breasts or thighs, cut into 4–5cm hunks

1 tbsp cumin seeds

1 tsp ground coriander

1 tsp paprika

a pinch of chilli powder

150ml orange juice

75ml olive oil, plus extra for glossing

a large handful of fresh coriander

1 tsp runny honey

2 onions, thinly sliced

2 red peppers, thinly sliced

1 courgette, cut into 2cm-thick batons

2 garlic cloves, finely minced

100g mixed salad leaves

100g alfalfa sprouts

2 ripe avocados, sliced

4 tbsp sunflower and/or pumpkin seeds, toasted

sea salt and freshly ground black pepper

Preheat the grill to high or your oven to 220°C/Gas 7. Place a grill pan or baking sheet on the top shelf to heat up.

Tumble the chicken into a small bowl. Mix the spices in a separate bowl. Dust half the spices over the meat and stir in well.

Place the orange juice, olive oil, a handful of coriander and the honey in a blender or food processor. Blitz until smooth and creamy. Alternatively, finely chop the coriander and pop it in a jam jar with the remaining ingredients. Secure the lid and shake well until mixed. Add a splash of the dressing over the meat, just enough to moisten. Mix well. Set aside to marinate.

Heat a large frying pan. Gloss with oil. Toss the onions, peppers and courgette batons into the pan. Sizzle over a medium-high heat until just tender and a little charred around the edges, 10–15 minutes.

Fold the garlic and remaining spice mix in and cook until fragrant. Season with salt and pepper, to taste, and remove from the heat.

Thread the meat onto skewers. Place on the warmed grill pan or baking sheet. Cook on the top shelf until golden and cooked through, about 5–7 minutes on each side. Gloss with a little of the remaining dressing once cooked.

Wash and dry the salad leaves and alfalfa sprouts. Toss with a good splash of the dressing, just enough to moisten.

Divide the veg between plates. Top with the mixed leaves and sprouts. Gently fold everything together. Dot the avocado slices over the top. Gloss with a little more dressing. Finish with the remaining herbs and the toasted seeds.

Variation: swap the chicken for quinoa. In a lidded frying pan, toast half a mug of quinoa for a second. Add half the spice mix and pour in 1 mug of water. Pop a lid on and cook over a low heat for 20 minutes or until all the water is absorbed. Let the quinoa cool a little before mixing with the onions, peppers and courgettes, then add to the leaves, avocados and seeds, followed by an extra gloss of dressing.

SOUK SALAD WITH SPICED AUBERGINES AND PISTACHIO YOGHURT

This makes an impressive party piece. Equally, it's a stunning packed lunch to tote into work to make your colleagues weep (pack the dressing in a lidded jam jar and dress just before serving). All the herbs, veg and spice packed into this pretty salad are hugely energising.

4 PORTIONS
PER SERVING

PREP 15 MINS
COOK 45 MINS
SERVES 4

4 handfuls of mixed salad leaves

2 handfuls of fresh herbs (use 2–3: mint, parsley, dill, coriander, chives, basil, tarragon, sorrel)

2 large handfuls of mixed seasonal veg●

a gloss of olive oil

2 pomegrananates

a handful of edible flowers (optional)

sea salt and ground pepper

FOR THE SPICED AUBERGINES
2 aubergines

1 garlic clove, chopped

a good gloss of olive oil

1 tbsp cumin seeds

1 tsp sweet paprika

1 tsp ground cloves

1 tsp ground cinnamon

a pinch of chilli powder

FOR THE PISTACHIO YOGHURT
6 tbsp shelled pistachios

a large handful of fresh mint

250g natural yoghurt

1–2 tsp olive oil

Preheat the oven to 220°C/Gas 7. Place a baking tray on the top shelf to heat up.

First, make the aubergines. Halve the aubergines lengthways. Make 1cm deep cuts on the diagonal, about 2cm apart. Repeat in the opposite direction, creating a criss-cross pattern. Rub the chopped garlic over the top. Dust with salt and pepper. Gloss with a generous drizzle of olive oil. Roast on the heated tray for 40 minutes until tender.

Mix up the aubergine spices. Dust over the cooked aubergine. Roast for another 5 minutes.

For the pistachio yoghurt, whizz the pistachios with the mint and yoghurt in a blender or food processor until smooth. Alternatively, grind the pistachios in a pestle and mortar, add the mint, pound it to a paste and whisk into the yoghurt. Season, to taste. Trickle in a little olive oil, as needed.

Clean your salad leaves. Mix in a large bowl with your herbs and seasonal veg. Sprinkle over a pinch of salt and pepper, gloss with a drop of olive oil and mix well.

Roll the pomegranates on a firm surface to loosen the seeds. Place a sieve over a bowl. Cut the pomegranates over the sieve so the juices are caught in the bowl. Pluck the seeds from the pomegranates: I do this by inverting the pomegranate halves; gently tease any stuck seeds out with your fingers. Remove any white pith from your pile of seeds.

Drizzle the pomegranate juice over the salad. Divide between plates. Dollop with some pistachio yoghurt. Plonk a spiced aubergine half on each salad. Finish with the pomegranate seeds and the edible flowers, if using. Serve the remaining yoghurt on the side.

● *My favourite mix is thinly sliced radishes (toss the leaves in with the salad leaves), thinly sliced cucumber rounds, tender purple sprouting broccoli florets, thinly sliced red onions (gently softened by placing them in a sieve and pouring boiling water over) and shavings of fennel (add the fronds to the herb mix).*

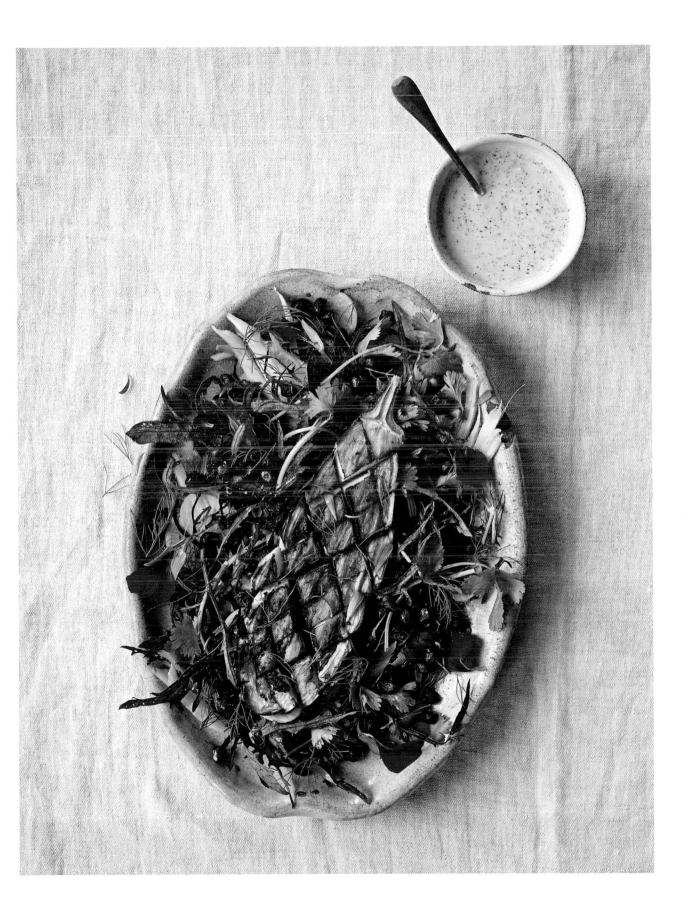

Rice

THE BASICS: When I'm tired, hungry and come home to a fridge full of odds and ends, rice is my saviour. I've tried all sorts of techniques for cooking rice and my favourite is the absorption method.

I tend to just grab a coffee mug, tea cup or any other available vessel. The ratio is 1 part rice to 2 parts water. A full mug (about 250g rice) will feed 4 people nicely, and to that I add 2 mugs of water. I toast rice instead of rinsing it. There's a moment of theatre to doing this, and it smells heavenly. After toasting, I pour the water over the warmed rice and pop a lid on. For white rice, cook for 12 minutes over low heat, then steam, lid-on but off the heat, for 5 minutes. For brown rice, I cook for 20 minutes, then steam for 10 minutes.

GORGEOUS GREEN INDIAN-SPICED RICE

 2 PORTIONS PER SERVING

PREP   10 MINS
COOK   30 MINS
SERVES 4

1 mug of brown basmati rice

a few glosses of olive oil

2 mugs of water

1 onion, finely diced

3 garlic cloves, finely chopped

1 tbsp freshly grated ginger

½ red chilli, finely chopped

1 tbsp cumin seeds

1 tsp fennel seeds

2 tsp ground turmeric

1 tsp ground coriander

1 head of broccoli

1 lemon or lime

a handful of fresh coriander and/or mint, chopped

a handful of cashews, toasted

sea salt and freshly ground black pepper

Heat a large lidded pan. Add the rice and a pinch of salt and toast for a moment. Add a gloss of olive oil and the water. Pop a lid on. Boil over a medium heat for 20 minutes or until all the water is absorbed, stirring occasionally.

While the rice cooks, heat a small frying pan for your onions. Add a gloss of oil and swirl in the chopped onions. Lower the heat and cook until glossy and tender, about 10 minutes. Fold in the garlic, ginger, chilli and other spices. Sizzle for a moment.

Chop the broccoli into tiny florets and thinly slice. You can use the stalk, too: just carve the tough outer skin and thinly slice or dice.

Once the rice has cooked for 20 minutes, pile the broccoli on top. Replace the lid and lower the heat. Allow the rice and veg to steam for 5–10 minutes, or until the rice has absorbed all the water and the broccoli is tender but still verdant. Add more water during cooking, if needed.

Take the lid off the broccoli rice. Swirl the spiced onion mix through. Grate in a little lemon or lime zest and a good squeeze of juice. Taste. Adjust seasoning as needed. Finish with fresh herbs and toasted cashews. Delicious served with a dollop of natural or coconut yogurt.

JERK LAMB WITH SUNSHINE RICE AND A LITTLE SALAD

I let my 7-year-old son, Rory, take charge of our weekly market shopping. I give him a budget and a rough list: get meat, eggs, some green veg, some root veg . . . and off he goes. On one occasion he came back from the butcher's counter with a rack of lamb and had the genius idea of pairing it with jerk spices, which I think work better with lamb than with chicken. Partnered with this fruit- and veg-rich rice, it's a dream.

 3.5 PORTIONS PER SERVING

PREP 15 MINS
COOK 30 MINS
SERVES 4

2 tsp ground nutmeg

2 tsp ground cloves

2 tsp ground allspice

1 tbsp brown sugar

½ Scotch Bonnet or any red chilli, finely chopped

4 tbsp rum (or pineapple juice)

4 tbsp white wine vinegar

3 garlic cloves, finely minced

1 tsp fresh thyme leaves, plus extra to garnish

4 bay leaves

4–8 lamb cutlets

2 onions, thinly sliced

1 mug of brown basmati rice

2 mugs of water

a few glosses of olive oil

1 pineapple, cut into 2–3cm thick rings

½ a fennel bulb, thinly sliced

1 red pepper, thinly sliced

1 lime, halved

sea salt

In a bowl, mix the nutmeg, cloves, allspice, sugar, Scotch Bonnet, rum, vinegar, garlic, fresh thyme and bay together.

Nestle the lamb and onions in a dish. Pierce the lamb all over with a fork, then pour over the marinade. Massage in. Leave to marinate for 10 minutes, or longer if you can.

Heat a lidded pan and add the rice. Toast for a few seconds. Add a drizzle of oil and a pinch of salt. Pour in the water. Pop a lid on and cook for 20 minutes or until the rice has guzzled up all the water. Once done, remove from the heat, lid on, and steam until ready to serve.

Pop a large frying pan over a high heat and add a gloss of oil. Cook the pineapple rings in a single layer, in batches, until nicely bronzed on each side. Remove from the pan.

Add another gloss of oil to the pan. Cook the onions and lamb with the marinade. Remove the cutlets once nicely coloured on each side, and cooked to your liking. To see how pink the lamb is, peer into the centre of one cutlet using a knife and fork. Let the lamb rest while you cook the onions for a touch longer, until nicely softened. Once cooked, fold the onions through the rice and scatter a few fresh thyme leaves over.

Toss the fennel and red pepper together. Drizzle with a trickle of oil and squeeze over a good hit of lime juice.

Pile the onion rice onto plates. Top with the pineapple, and place the lamb alongside. Scatter a few more thyme leaves over the top. Place the fennel and red pepper salad in the centre of the table and get stuck in.

Variation: to make this vegan, swap the lamb for sweet potato wedges, roasted or pan fried in the spices until crisp on the outside and tender in the middle.

NOTE: Speed things up by marinating the lamb in the morning or the night before. Then it's a doddle to throw together.

CHARD DOLMADES WITH WILD RICE, GRAPES, FETA AND FENNEL WITH LITTLE FISH

Grapes and fennel seeds are a match made in heaven. This is a gorgeous autumnal dish and the perfect way to make a mound of chard leaves look really exciting.

 2 PORTIONS PER SERVING

PREP 10 MINS
COOK 35 MINS
SERVES 4

100g wild rice

300g black or red seedless grapes, halved

1 fennel bulb, cut into 1cm dice

2 tsp fennel seeds, toasted

a good pinch of chilli flakes or finely chopped fresh chilli (more or less, to taste)

zest and juice of 1 lemon

100g feta, crumbled

a drizzle of olive oil

2 large handfuls of fresh mint, parsley and/or basil

8 large chard leaves (about 120g)

sea salt and freshly ground black pepper

FOR THE FISH
300g whole sprats or 8 sardine fillets

1 lemon

6 fresh rosemary sprigs

a pinch of chilli flakes or a thinly sliced red chilli

a gloss of olive oil

Preheat the oven grill to high or oven to 220°C/Gas 7.

Place a pan of boiling water on the hob. Add the rice. Pop a lid on and simmer over a medium-low heat for 35 minutes, or until tender. Some of the grains will have split open which is a sign it's done. Drain off the excess water.

Arrange the sprats or sardines in a large roasting dish. Season well and grate a little lemon zest over. Slice the lemon and tuck the slices and rosemary sprigs in amongst the sardines. Scatter the chilli over and gloss with oil. Place under the grill or in the oven for 10 minutes, or until the fish are golden and crisp.

Mix the cooked rice with the halved grapes, diced fennel, toasted fennel seeds, chilli, lemon zest and a squeeze of juice, and the feta. Season to taste. Drizzle with a little oil and scatter over a good heap of fresh herbs, gently folding them through.

Wash and dry the chard leaves. Serve them on the side for people to fill; just heap a mound of the salad in the centre and then fold the sides in before rolling into a little parcel.

Serve with the warm fish.

NOTE: For a super healthy option, you can sprout your wild rice. This involves soaking your wild rice in cold water for 3 days, rinsing the rice and changing the water each day. You can tell when it's ready to eat as the grain will be tender, but with a little nuttiness like a fresh walnut, and some of them will start to 'bloom' or split open and curl up a little.

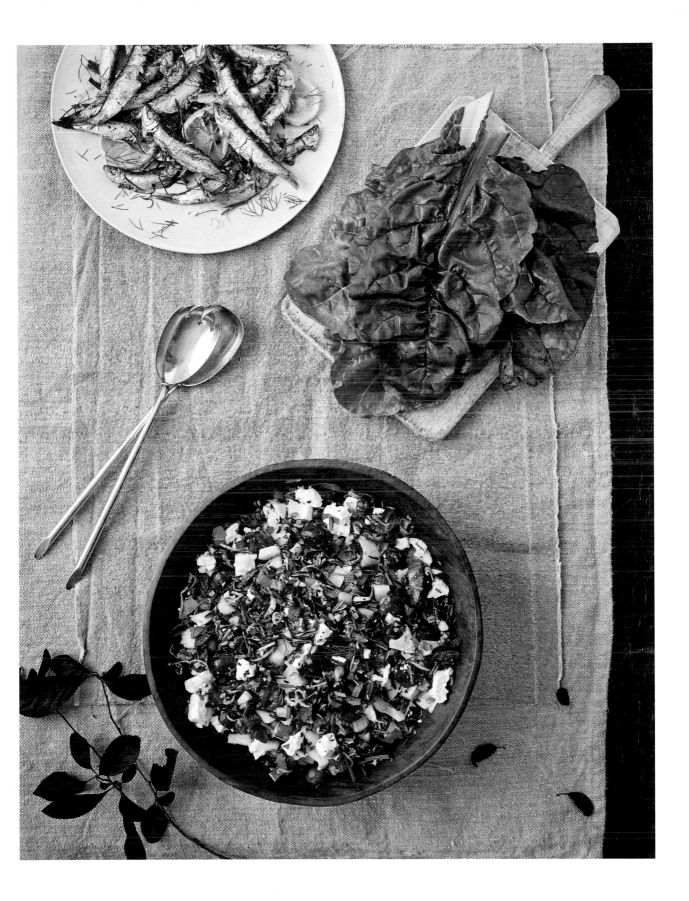

SPANISH RICE WITH ROASTED CAULIFLOWER AND MARCONA ALMONDS

This is a veg-laden nod to paella but is in no way authentic. By no means does that take away from its absolute deliciousness.

 2.5 PORTIONS PER SERVING

PREP 10 MINS
COOK 35 MINS
SERVES 4

a pinch of saffron (optional)

1 mug of brown basmati rice

a few glugs of olive oil

2 mugs of hot chicken or veg stock

1 large cauliflower, cut into florets

2 red peppers, cut into 2cm-thick slices (seeds and stem discarded) •

2 onions, sliced

1 whole bulb of garlic

3 tbsp tomato purée

2 tsp paprika (use sweet, smoked paprika, if possible)

a pinch of chilli powder

zest and juice of 1 lemon

a large handful of fresh parsley, finely chopped

a large handful of Marcona or toasted plain almonds

sea salt and freshly ground black pepper

Preheat the oven to 220°C/Gas 7. Pop a large roasting tray in the oven to heat.

Place the saffron in a little cup with 2 tablespoons of boiling water, if using. Stir and set aside.

Heat a pan with a lid and add the rice and a pinch of salt. Toast for a moment, add a drizzle of oil and pour in the stock. Bring to the boil. Reduce the heat, pop a lid on and cook for 20 minutes, or until all the water's absorbed. Once cooked, let it steam off the heat, lid on, for a further 5 minutes.

Toss the cauliflower florets, red pepper and onions into a bowl. Gloss with oil, season and mix well. Slice the pointy top off your garlic bulb, just exposing the cloves. Tumble the veg and garlic onto the warmed roasting tray, shake to distribute evenly, and add a little more oil, if needed. Roast for 25 minutes, or until the veg is tender and has bronzed a little.

Once your rice is cooked, fluff it with a fork, then swirl in the saffron and soaking liquid along with the tomato purée, paprika and chilli powder. Add the lemon zest and juice, taste, and adjust the seasoning to your liking.

Once the veg is done, squeeze out the garlic cloves (like toothpaste) into the rice. Fold through, along with half the parsley. Gently mix your veg through and finish with an extra spritz of lemon juice, the remaining parsley and the almonds.

> • *Swap the fresh red pepper for a small jar of piquillo peppers, torn into ribbons. Just fold them through the rice when you add the roasted cauliflower.*

SENEGALESE PEANUT RICE WITH STICKY GINGER PUMPKIN

When we first met, my husband and I had an A-to-Z culinary adventure around London's ethnic restaurants, inspired by our first date in an Afghan restaurant. We must have been exposed to something like this recipe along the way. These flavour combos, textures and tastes are lodged in my memory, and are very much Senegalese in style, with peanuts, spice, coconut and squash. After a little playing around in the kitchen, I arrived at the exact dish I had been holding in my head. It's deeply satisfying.

 3 PORTIONS
PER SERVING

PREP   10 MINS
COOK   30 MINS
SERVES   4

1 mug of brown basmati rice

2 mugs of water

a gloss of oil (coconut, olive or ghee)

750g–1kg pumpkin or squash, cut into 6 x 2cm chunks

3 garlic cloves, finely chopped

a good pinch of chilli flakes•

2 tbsp freshly grated ginger

4 tbsp crunchy peanut butter

1 tbsp ground turmeric or 2 tbsp freshly grated

300ml coconut milk

100g baby spinach leaves

a handful of fresh parsley or coriander leaves

sea salt and freshly ground black pepper

Heat a lidded pan and add the rice and a pinch of salt. Toast for a moment, then add a drizzle of oil and pour in the water. Simmer for 20 minutes with the lid on, or until the rice has absorbed all the water. Remove from the heat, lid on, and let the rice steam for 5 minutes.

While the rice is cooking, heat a large, lidded frying pan and add a good gloss of oil, enough to generously coat the pan. Add the pumpkin chunks and a pinch of salt. Cook in batches, if necessary, as you don't want to overcrowd the pan. Let the pumpkin sizzle for a bit, then pop on a lid and cook until tender, 10–15 minutes.

Remove the lid, crank up the heat and add half the garlic, chilli and ginger. Continue to cook until the squash is sticky, soft and a touch golden. Taste, adjust the seasoning to suit and remove from the heat.

Remove the lid from the rice. Swirl in the peanut butter, turmeric and the remaining garlic, ginger and chilli. Fold in the coconut milk. Warm over a medium heat to let it cook into the rice a little. The rice should have a slightly loose, risotto-like texture. Add a little more coconut milk or water to achieve this, if necessary.

Swirl in the spinach. Cook for just a second, long enough to soften the leaves. Season, to taste.

Pile the rice on plates. Top with the pumpkin and a dash of herbs and/or chilli flakes, to garnish.

> • *If you can get a hold of some smoky chipotle chillies use them in place of the chilli flakes. Just chop the dried chillies to make your own flakes. Add a pinch at a time until you get the right level of heat for you.*

Pasta

THE BASICS: When you're in a rush, or when you're trying to sneak some veg into your children, pasta is the magic word. For the most part, I opt for wholegrain pasta. I find it has a richer, nuttier flavour and more grip for your sauce. Once cooked and dressed, wholegrain sceptics hardly notice the difference; it's very subtle, but has enormous benefits health-wise.

Rub a little oil into the bottom of the pan before cooking. If I'm cooking a small pasta shape, I'll toss the pasta in and coat in the oil before adding the water. This helps the pasta from sticking together or to the bottom of the pan. For spaghetti, tagliatelle and other long strands of pasta, I gloss the bottom of the pot with oil, add the water and then the pasta. Stir a few times throughout cooking too, to help prevent the dreaded clumping or stuck-to-the-bottom strands. When draining the pasta, always keep a tablespoon or two of the cooking water to mix with the sauce.

SUMMER TOMATO AND SEED PENNE

Camp stove and bottle of water to hand, this is the sort of thing you can make on your allotment or in your garden on a summer's eve. But even with some shop-bought tomatoes, indoors, on a rainy day, it's a heavenly, super-speedy supper.

3 PORTIONS PER SERVING

PREP   5 MINS
COOK   15 MINS
SERVES 4

a few glosses of olive oil

300g penne pasta

1kg cherry tomatoes, halved or quartered if on the larger side

1 garlic clove, finely chopped

4 tbsp mixed seeds (pumpkin, sunflower and/or poppy seeds), toasted

a large handful of fresh herbs (basil, parsley, chervil, chives), torn

sea salt and freshly ground black pepper

Gloss a large saucepan with a little oil. Fill with water, add a pinch of sea salt and bring to the boil. Plunge the pasta in. Cook according to packet instructions, typically 12 minutes for perfect al dente.

While the pasta is cooking, tumble the halved/quartered tomatoes and the garlic into a bowl with a pinch of salt and pepper. Get your hands in there and give it a good mix, until all the juices are released from the tomatoes.

Drain the pasta. Gloss with a little olive oil and toss in the tomatoes and most of the seeds, keeping back a few to sprinkle over the top. Mix well.

Fold in most of the herbs, again leaving a few to scatter on top. Plate up, adding a finishing touch of seeds and herbs.

HAZELNUTTY FAIRY CABBAGE PASTA

The lovely Steven Lamb from River Cottage changed my relationship with Brussels sprouts forever when he called them fairy cabbages; that's how he's managed to get his daughters to love the Marmite of veg. My son, at age 7, however, wasn't impressed when I told him we were having fairy cabbages for dinner. No matter what you call them, this dish is a game-changer for sprout haters, miles away from the over-boiled mush that's put many a generation off this lovely veg.

 PORTIONS PER SERVING

PREP   15 MINS
COOK   15 MINS
SERVES 4

a few glosses of olive oil

300g pasta (a smallish, shell-like shape works best)

500g small Brussels sprouts, or use halved or quartered larger sprouts

a large handful of hazelnuts

1 garlic clove, finely minced

a pinch of chilli flakes or finely chopped red chilli

a small knob of butter

zest and juice of 1 lemon

freshly grated Parmesan, to serve

sea salt and freshly ground black pepper

Gloss a large saucepan with a little oil. Fill with water, add a pinch of sea salt, and bring to the boil. Plunge the pasta in. Cook according to packet instructions, typically 12 minutes for perfect al dente.

While the pasta is cooking, heat a large frying pan. Add the sprouts and a pinch of salt and pepper. Cook them in the hot pan with no oil for a few moments, until they're all toasty.

Add a gloss of oil and the hazelnuts. Shake the pan to toss them through the oil. Once the sprouts are bright green and nutty tasting (try one) and the nuts are fragrant and toasty, toss in the garlic, chilli and a drop more oil, if needed. Fold it through until softened.

Drain the pasta. Add to the sprouts along with a knob of butter or a little extra oil. Add the lemon zest and a good hit of juice. Taste, and adjust the seasoning to your liking. Finish with a grating of Parmesan or extra chilli, if you like.

RADICCHIO PASTA RAGS WITH BALSAMIC, PINE NUTS AND SAUSAGE CRUMBS

I love radicchio. It's one of the most beautiful vegetables – the rose of the cabbage patch. In this dish especially, it's an absolute joy to eat.

2 PORTIONS
PER SERVING

PREP   10 MINS
COOK   15 MINS
SERVES 4

a few glosses of olive oil

1 large red onion, thinly sliced

300g dried lasagne sheets, broken into largish pieces●

3–4 good-quality pork sausages

1 large or 2 small heads of radicchio, quartered and thinly sliced

3 garlic cloves, finely minced

4 tbsp balsamic vinegar

1 sprig of fresh rosemary, leaves finely chopped, or a good pinch of dried rosemary

a pinch of chilli powder

a small knob of butter

4 tbsp pine nuts

a small handful of fresh parsley, finely chopped

sea salt and freshly ground black pepper

Heat a large frying pan and add a gloss of oil. Tumble the sliced onion into the pan, lower the heat and cook until meltingly tender.

While the onions are cooking, gloss a large saucepan with a little oil. Fill with water, add a pinch of sea salt and bring to the boil. Plunge the pasta in. Cook according to packet instructions, typically 12 minutes for perfect al dente, but test during cooking.

Heat another frying pan for the sausages. Squeeze the meat from the sausage casings and place in the hot pan, breaking it up into small pieces as it cooks. You could fry this with the onions if you prefer, but I like cooking it separately as it lends more texture and a layering of flavours to the final dish.

Quarter the radicchio and cut into thin ribbons, discarding the tough inner white core. Add the radicchio ribbons and garlic to the onions with a good hit of freshly ground pepper. Fold through with about 2–3 tablespoons of water, enough to just moisten.

When the radicchio is tender and the water's been guzzled up, add the balsamic vinegar, rosemary and a pinch of chilli powder. Let the balsamic cook into the radicchio. Remove from the heat.

Drain the pasta, toss with a little butter or oil and add to the radicchio.

Add the pine nuts to the sausage meat and cook until golden.

Pile the radicchio pasta rags onto plates. Scatter over the sausage crumbs and toasted pine nuts and finish with a little parsley.

● *If you don't have lasagne sheets, swap for spaghetti or your favourite pasta.*

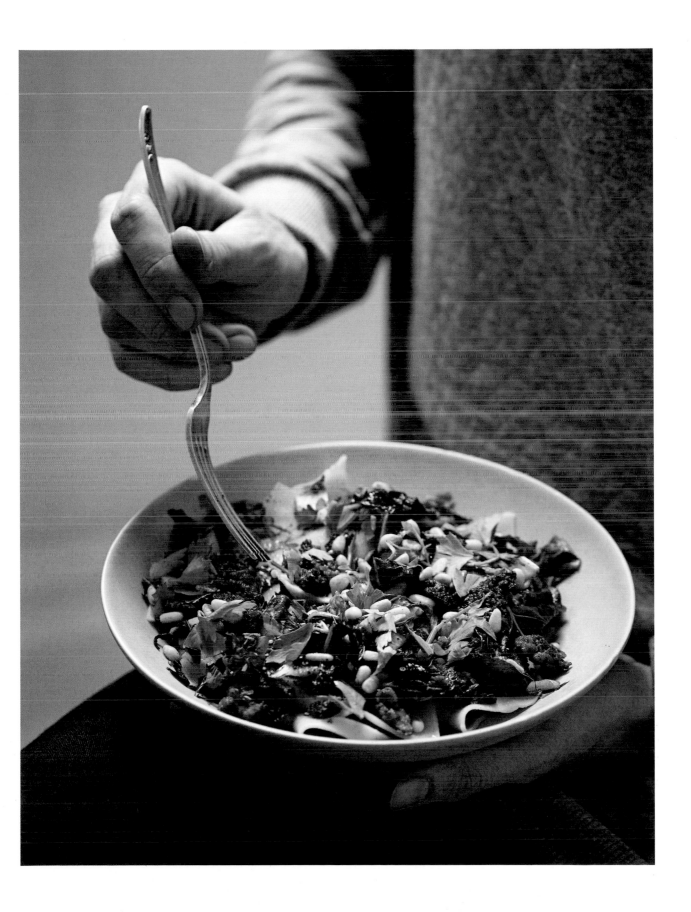

ESPRESSO MUSHROOMS WITH TAGLIATELLE

A friend of mine grows mushrooms in coffee, and his company, Espresso Mushrooms, gave me the idea for this pairing. The coffee is subtle, so even if you're not a fan, but you love mushrooms, I think you'll like this dish as it completely elevates their rich, earthy, mesmerising flavour.

 3 PORTIONS
PER SERVING

PREP   15 MINS
COOK   15 MINS
SERVES 4

a few glosses of olive oil

300g tagliatelle (or your favourite pasta shape)

1kg mushrooms, thinly sliced or torn (I use chestnut, but any will work)

2 garlic cloves, finely minced

200ml freshly brewed black coffee

100ml mascarpone or cream (optional)

a large handful of walnuts, roughly chopped and toasted

a little fresh parsley or chervil (optional)

sea salt and freshly ground black pepper

Gloss a large pan with a little oil. Fill with water, add a pinch of sea salt and bring to the boil. Plunge the pasta in. Cook according to the packet instructions, typically 12 minutes for perfect al dente.

Heat a large frying pan and add a splash of olive oil, enough to coat the bottom of the pan. Add the mushrooms and sizzle with a pinch of salt and a good hit of pepper (not just to season but to give it a bit of a kick) until nicely golden. Swirl the garlic through the mushrooms and cook for a moment. Keep the pan over a high heat and pour in the coffee. Let the mushrooms drink it up until there's only a splash of liquid left in the pan.

Drain the pasta, reserving 2 tablespoons of the cooking water.

Take the mushrooms off the heat and swirl in the mascarpone or cream. Taste, adjust the seasoning to taste, and add more cream or coffee, if desired. Toss with the warm pasta, swirling in a little of the cooking liquid, if needed. Scatter over the walnuts and herbs, and serve.

Variation: for a vegan/dairy-free/diet option, skip the cream and add a little more coffee instead of the cooking liquid.

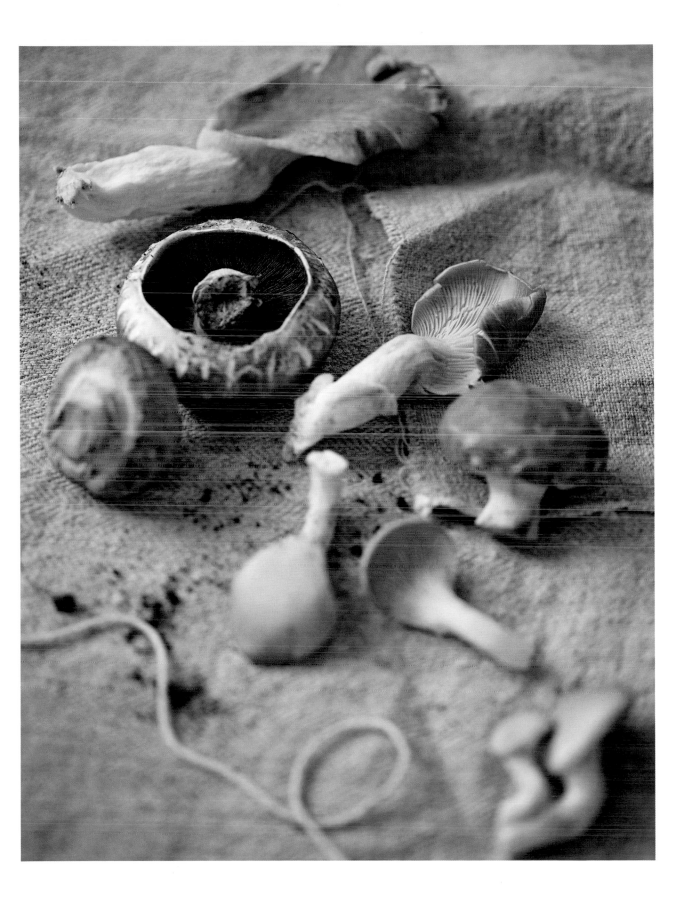

WILD SPRING SPAGHETTI

I love foraging, and gather wild greens whenever I can. My favourite flush of greens comes in spring when wild garlic, nettles and dandelion greens are everywhere. But all manner of wild greens would work a treat in this dish: ground elder, Jack-by-the-Hedge, or you could just use spinach or kale.

 2 PORTIONS
PER SERVING

PREP   10 MINS
COOK   25 MINS
SERVES 4

a gloss of olive oil

300g spaghetti (or your favourite pasta shape)

400g wild greens, cleaned and roughly chopped

4 egg yolks

100ml cream or crème fraîche

50g Parmesan or similar cheese, grated

1 garlic clove, finely minced (if your greens don't include wild garlic)

3–4 tbsp pine nuts, toasted (optional)

sea salt and freshly ground black pepper

Gloss a large saucepan with a little oil. Fill with water, add a pinch of salt and bring to the boil. Plunge the pasta in. Cook according to packet instructions, typically 12 minutes for perfect al dente.

Place the wild greens in a sieve and pour over enough boiling water to fully dampen and lightly cook them. Rinse under cold water, then gently squeeze out any excess water. Set aside.

Whisk the egg yolks, cream and Parmesan together until well mixed.

Drain the pasta, reserving 3–4 tablespoons of the cooking water. Pop it back in the pan. Swirl the egg mixture through the warm pasta, along with the garlic, if using. Place over a low heat to thicken it a little, stirring often. If it's looking too thick, swirl in the reserved cooking water.

Fold the greens through the saucy pasta. Add a good hit of black pepper. Taste, and adjust the seasoning, as needed. Pile onto plates. Finish with toasted pinenuts, if you've got them.

Delicious with griddled asparagus on the side in spring; in winter I'd pair it with roasted squash wedges.

Noodles

THE BASICS: I love noodles – you can pack heaps of veg into them, bunging them into a soup or tossing them through a stir fry. For those on a gluten-free diet, there's an array of wheat-free options, and they're the perfect staple item for vegans.

Typically noodles take just minutes to cook. The key is to follow the instructions on the packet, as the style, thickness and type of grain used to make the noodle dictate how long they take to cook. I like to gloss the bottom of my pan with a little oil to stop the noodles sticking, then add a pinch of salt to the water. Once cooked, rinsing the noodles under cold water for a few seconds will keep them from sticking together. Then toss with a little oil.

I've kept all these recipes Asian-themed as I can't get enough chilli, ginger, garlic, soy sauce and curry spice. It's all those great umami flavours that make for dishes you crave and dream about. However, you could go fusion and toss your noodles with Middle Eastern or even Italian flavours – have a play with the ingredients you love and come up with creations of your own.

CARROT AND STAR ANISE

This is one of my turn-to dishes when I would really rather not cook. It's so simple and deliciously satisfying that it makes me happy I didn't dine out.

PORTIONS PER SERVING

PREP   5 MINS
COOK   10 MINS
SERVES 4

300g buckwheat soba (or other) noodles

4 star anise (or 1 cinnamon stick and 4 cloves)

1–2 tbsp oil

12 spring onions, thinly sliced on the diagonal

4 good-sized carrots, coarsely grated

a pinch of chilli flakes, to taste

a few shakes of soy sauce

1 lime (optional)

100g cashew nuts, toasted

a handful of fresh coriander, parsley or basil, chopped, to serve

sea salt

Put the noodles in an oiled frying pan with the star anise and pour boiling water over them. Add a pinch of salt, stir to untangle the noodles and simmer for around 4 minutes (or according to packet instructions). Taste a noodle to ensure they're fully soft, then drain and rinse under cold water. Toss with a little more oil.

Pop the empty frying pan back on the heat and crank the heat up to high. Add a little oil, lower the heat and add the spring onions. Sizzle until they're soft and starting to crisp.

Add the carrots and a pinch of chilli to the pan with the onions. Pluck the star anise from the noodles and add to the pan. Sizzle until the carrots are soft and a little coloured around the edges. Add more oil, if needed.

Remove from the heat and fold the noodles through. Add a good hit of soy sauce, taste, and tweak the seasoning as needed. Divide between plates and finish with a squeeze of lime juice, toasted cashews, a little more chilli (if desired) and fresh herbs.

CHINESE SEAWEED

If you're not too sure about kale, this might just change your mind. It's sweet, salty and crispy, and a dream with a tangle of soy-sauce-glossed noodles.

 2 PORTIONS
PER SERVING

PREP   10 MINS
COOK   10 MINS
SERVES 4

a good splash of oil
  (rapeseed, coconut,
  olive oil)

400g kale or cavolo nero,
  finely chopped

2 tsp caster or coconut palm
  sugar

1 large garlic clove, finely
  minced

1 tsp dried chilli flakes
  (more or less, to taste)

300g rice noodles
  (vermicelli are the best)

a few shakes of soy sauce

sea salt

Preheat the oven to 220°C/Gas 7. Place a large baking sheet on the top shelf to heat up.

Heat a large frying pan and add enough oil to coat the pan. Toss in the kale with a good pinch of sea salt and sugar. Sizzle over a medium-high heat until it starts to crisp up. Fold the garlic and chilli flakes through. Remove from the heat.

Arrange the kale on the hot baking sheet in a single layer. Cook for around 3–5 minutes until it crisps up further. Remove from the oven and set aside; it will continue to crisp up.

Meanwhile, put the noodles in the empty frying pan and pour boiling water over them. Add a pinch of salt, stir to untangle the noodles and simmer for a minute or two (or according to packet instructions). Taste a noodle to ensure they're fully soft, then drain and rinse under cold water. Toss with a little more oil.

Tumble the noodles back into the frying pan. Add a few shakes of soy sauce. Scatter the crispy kale over the top, taste, and add more soy or chilli, if needed. Divide the noodles between plates and tuck in.

Delicious on their own as a simple main or serve with golden, pan-fried scallops or grilled mackerel.

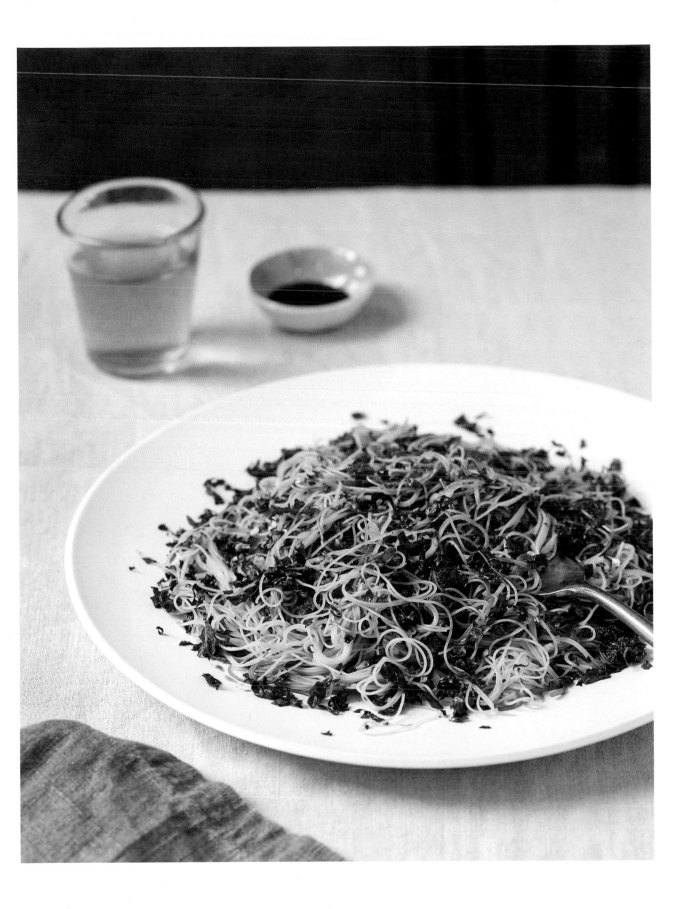

MISO GINGER TOMATO SOBA WITH JAPANESE STEAK

Tomato with ginger and miso is another of my favourite food trios. If you can get hold of some shisho leaves, it makes this dish extra stunning, but if not, snipped chives and chive flowers work a treat both visually and taste-wise.

 3.5 PORTIONS PER SERVING

PREP 10 MINS
COOK 15 MINS
SERVES 4

2 sirloin steaks

4 tbsp soy sauce

1 tbsp runny honey

3 garlic cloves, finely minced

½ red chilli, finely minced (more or less, to taste)

1 tbsp freshly grated ginger

1kg cherry tomatoes, halved

250g spring onions, thinly sliced

1 tbsp miso paste

3–4 tbsp hot water

200g buckwheat soba (or other) noodles

a few glosses of olive oil

sea salt and freshly ground black pepper

a few shisho leaves or snipped chives and chive flowers, to garnish (optional)

Bring the steaks to room temperature. Mix half the soy sauce with the honey, half the garlic and half the chilli, then pour over the steaks. Use a fork to pierce your steak all over, on both sides. This tenderises the meat and helps the marinade penetrate it.

Mix the remaining garlic and chilli with the ginger, tomatoes and spring onions. Whisk the miso paste and hot water until smooth.

Put the noodles in an oiled frying pan and pour boiling water over them. Add a pinch of salt, stir to untangle the noodles and simmer for around 4–7 minutes (or according to packet instructions). Taste a noodle to ensure they're fully soft, then drain and rinse under cold water. Toss with a little more oil.

Heat another frying pan for the steaks. Add a gloss of oil to the marinated steaks and transfer them to the hot pan. Cook for at least a minute before flipping; you'll see them starting to colour up on the side. Season the cooked side.

Once the steaks are nicely coloured on each side, test to ensure they're cooked to your liking. Pinch your index finger and thumb together, then feel the fleshy bit of your hand below your thumb. Press your finger on the steak – if it feels the same, the steak is rare. (Thumb to middle finger = medium rare; thumb to ring finger = medium well; thumb to little finger = well-done.)

If your steak has a fatty rind, you can crisp it up by holding the steak upright with tongs and pressing the fatty rind into the pan until nicely golden and crisp. Remove the steaks from the pan and set aside to rest.

Return the frying pan to the heat and tumble the tomatoes and spring onions into the pan. Let them colour up and soften slightly, moving them around the pan from time to time, but not too often.

Add the noodles to the pan and drizzle the miso paste over. Let it cook for a moment to warm through, then pile onto plates.

Thinly slice the steak and drape over the top or serve alongside. Finish with a pinch of shiso or snipped chives and chive flowers, or any soft herbs like parsley or basil.

CURRIED EGG-FRIED NOODLES

 4 PORTIONS
PER SERVING

PREP 15 MINS
COOK 20 MINS
SERVES 4

8 spring onions, 2 leeks or 1 large onion

150g rice or buckwheat noodles

a gloss of sesame or other oil (coconut, olive or rapeseed)

1kg selection seasonal veg•

1 thumb-sized piece of fresh ginger, peeled and finely chopped

2 garlic cloves, finely chopped

1–2 tbsp curry powder

200ml water

4 eggs, whisked

a splash of soy sauce, to finish

a pinch of fresh chilli slices or chilli flakes, to finish

a handful of fresh parsley or coriander, roughly chopped

sea salt

a handful of crushed, salted peanuts

Get some water on the boil. Cut your veg into bite-sized chunks. Slice the spring onions or leeks at the diagonal into chunks or thinly slice the onion.

Place the rice noodles in a large frying pan. Gloss with oil. Add a pinch of sea salt. Pour boiling water over them. Let them simmer until just tender, about 4 minutes (or according to pack instructions).

Drain. Rinse under cold water. Gloss with a little more oil.

Use the same frying pan to cook your veg. Place it over a high heat. Once smoking hot, add your veg and the onions/leeks but no oil. Let the veg griddle and toast in the pan until softened and charring a little around the edges.

Swirl in the ginger, garlic and curry powder, start with 1 tablespoon and add more to bolster flavour and colour, as needed. Pour in the water. Mix to help it swirl the curry spices around the pan. Fold in your noodles. Once the water is gone, push your veg to one side of the pan.

Add a little gloss of oil to the bare side of the pan. Add your whisked eggs. Let them cook through, stirring them (but keeping them separate from the veg and noodles) until set and scrambled. Fold the eggs through the noodles and veg. Taste. Add more curry powder, a hit of salt or soy sauce and a hit of chilli to suit your tastebuds.

Pile onto plates. Finish with a scattering of fresh herbs and extra chilli.

> • *One of my favourite combos is 2 carrots, 1 red pepper, 1 small or ½ large bulb of fennel and a bundle of purple sprouting or regular broccoli but use whatever you've got to hand. Other faves: shredded cabbage or kale or matchsticks of black radish, kohlrabi and courgettes.*

ASPARAGUS CRAB NOODLES WITH LEMON CHILLI DRESSING

Once you've got the asparagus in ribbons, this dish is super-quick to make. It is well worth having the asparagus ribbons as they cook perfectly in seconds and have a gorgeous texture. If you're in a rush, thinly slice your asparagus into rounds instead, leaving the tips chunky.

 2.5 PORTIONS PER SERVING

PREP 20 MINS
COOK 10 MINS
SERVES 4

650g asparagus

zest and juice of 1 lemon (or orange, lime or ponzu – or a combo)

4 tbsp olive oil or melted coconut oil, plus extra for greasing

1 tbsp soy sauce

½ a red chilli, more or less to taste

1 small garlic clove, finely minced

250g rice or buckwheat noodles

150g spring onions, thinly sliced

200g fresh crab meat (white or a 50: 50 mix of brown and white)

a pinch of finely ground Szechuan peppercorns (optional)

a handful of fresh chervil, parsley, basil and/or coriander

sea salt and freshly ground black pepper

Snap the woody ends from the base of the asparagus (you can feel the woody bits with your fingers). Hold the asparagus by the tip with one hand and use the other hand to glide a veg peeler along the stalk, creating ribbons. Holding your spear at the edge of a cutting board helps as well. The middle bits will be a bit chunky but this adds to the texture and flavour of the dish.

Once the ribbons are done, whisk the citrus zest and 4 tablespoons of juice with the oil, soy sauce, chilli and garlic.

Put the noodles in an oiled frying pan and pour boiling water over them. Add a pinch of salt, stir to untangle the noodles and simmer for 4 minutes (or according to packet instructions). Add the asparagus ribbons and sliced spring onions to your noodles 30 seconds before you take them off the heat. Swirl through the boiling water, then drain everything.

While the noodles are cooking, add a good pinch of salt and pepper to the crab meat.

Toss the warm asparagus noodles with the crab and dressing. Season with salt and pepper to taste. Dust a pinch of Szechuan pepper over, too, if you like. Taste, and adjust seasoning, adding more citrus zest, juice and chilli, if needed. Plate up and finish with a scattering of fresh herbs. Serve straight away or chill and eat cold. A lovely dish for a spring picnic.

Variation: omit the rice/wheat noodles and simply mix the asparagus ribbons with the crab and dressing for a lighter, carb-free meal.

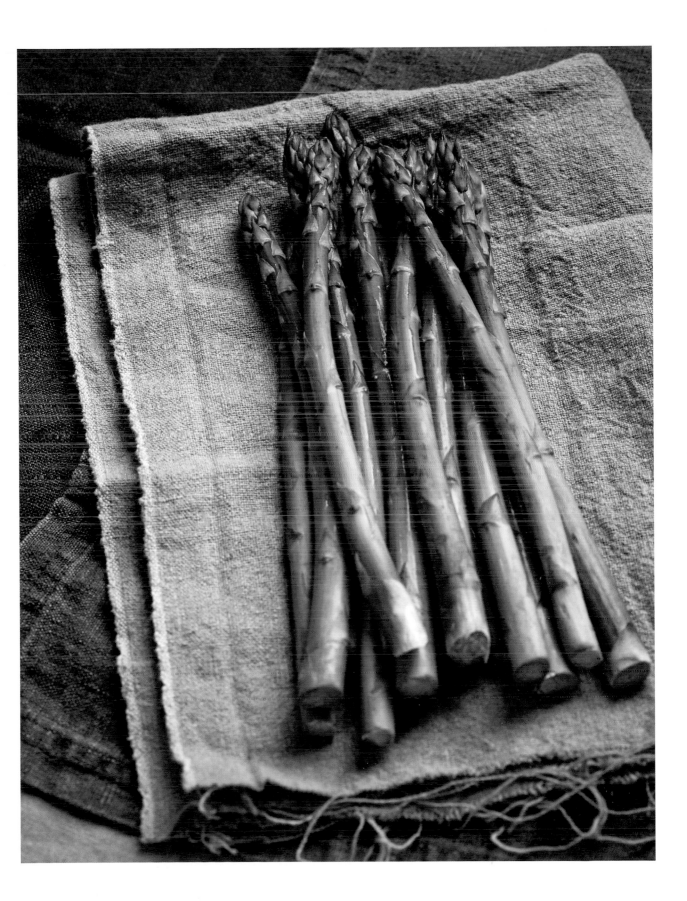

Curries

THE BASICS: I grew up in Texas, where curry is not something you come across often. In fact, I didn't eat my first curry until I was 20, when I was hooked with my first bite.

The starting point of pretty much every curry is the culinary trinity of garlic, ginger and chilli. Next on the list is a medley of spices. I think it's fun to pick one or two key spices to star in a curry, be it cinnamon, cardamom, fresh turmeric and so forth. Tomatoes and coconut milk also play a huge role in most curries. You can marry both, or allow one to feature on its own. Or skip both and have a dry curry of fried spices and veg with water or stock. There are no set rules. So throw out the rule books out and turn your kitchen into a den of spice alchemy.

COCONUT CABBAGE CURRY

I have to admit, cabbage used to be my least-loved veg, but then this dish was born. Not only does it shift an entire bowling-ball-sized brassica from your fridge, it also fills you up with good-for-you comfort food.

 PORTIONS PER SERVING

PREP   10 MINS
COOK   20 MINS
SERVES 4

a few splashes of olive oil

1 onion, finely chopped

3 garlic cloves, chopped

1 red chilli, finely chopped

2 tbsp freshly grated ginger

1 cinnamon stick or a pinch
    of ground cinnamon

3 bay leaves (optional)

2 tsp cumin seeds

2 tsp ground turmeric

1 cabbage, finely shredded

250ml water

400g tin of coconut milk

zest and juice of 1 lime

a handful of fresh coriander
    or parsley, chopped

a large handful of cashews,
    toasted

sea salt and freshly ground
    black pepper

Heat a wok or a large frying pan and add a splash of oil. Tumble in the onion and a pinch of salt, lower the heat and fry until tender, stirring often. Mix in the garlic, chilli and ginger and cook for a moment until softened. Add the cinnamon, bay and all the remaining spices, stir, and cook until fragrant.

Fold the cabbage through and turn up the heat. Add the water and let it sizzle and reduce right down, until it's almost evaporated. Stir the cabbage as it cooks.

Once the water's gone, pour in the coconut milk, stir, and cook until thickened slightly. Add a little lime zest and a squeeze of juice. Taste, and adjust the seasoning if needed. Scatter over the fresh coriander and toasted cashews and serve with rice.

SUMMER TOMATO AND BEAN

For gardeners, this is the dish to make at the end of August or early September when the sun is shining and the garden's full of sun-drenched tomatoes and bundles of beans. But even if you don't have a garden of your own, this dish is a dream to make and eat as it's packed full of fresh ingredients. The curry is just as beautiful without the meat, or with leftover roast lamb or raw nuggets of fish (placed in the broth to gently cook though).

 4 PORTIONS FOR EVERY 4 CHUNKS OF SQUASH

PREP 10 MINS
COOK 25 MINS
SERVES 4

1kg cherry tomatoes

1 chilli

2 tbsp freshly grated ginger

4 garlic cloves

a gloss of olive oil

2 onions, thinly sliced

2 cinnamon sticks

10 whole cloves

¼ tsp freshly ground black pepper

1 tsp ground turmeric

1 tbsp curry leaves

400g tin of coconut milk

250g diced chicken breast or boneless thigh/leg meat

250g French beans, topped and tailed

a handful of fresh chives, coriander, basil and/or parsley, chopped

sea salt

Place half the tomatoes in a blender or food processor. Halve the chilli lengthways, scrape out the seeds and membrane (save the seeds to plant), and add to the blender/food processor with the ginger and garlic. Purée until smooth.

Cut the remaining tomatoes in half and set aside.

Heat a large saucepan and add a gloss of oil. Tumble in the sliced onions with a pinch of salt. Cook over a low heat until glossy and tender. Swirl in the cinnamon, cloves, black pepper, turmeric and curry leaves. Add the halved tomatoes, cut side-down. Let them cook for a few minutes to soften and colour up a bit. Pour in the puréed tomatoes and cook until the mixture has reduced down slightly, about 5 minutes. Add the coconut milk, chicken and beans. Let the curry bubble away for 15 minutes.

Taste the curry and adjust the seasoning, to taste. Finish with a scattering of fresh herbs and pair with warm cumin chana dosas (see below).

CUMIN CHANA DOSA

Mix 150g plain white flour with 150g chickpea (gram) flour in a large bowl. Swirl in ½ tsp sea salt, ½ tsp bicarbonate of soda and 2 tsp cumin seeds. Whisk in 400ml warm water until you have a smooth batter the consistency of single cream. Add more flour or water, if needed, to achieve this. Heat a large frying pan. Brush with oil, coating the inside of your pan. Give the batter a final whisk. Pour in the batter to form a circle half as big as the pan, then swirl it around to stretch the circle out toward the sides. Once the batter is cooked and crispy around the edges and has bubbles setting toward the centre, use a spatula to flip it. Gloss the top with oil, butter or ghee. Place on a plate covered by another plate to keep the cooked dosas soft and warm while you repeat with the remaining batter.

CHLOE CHICKPEAS WITH SPICED LAMB SKEWERS AND HERB YOGHURT

This simple but lovely North Indian curry is the perfect storecupboard supper partnered with spice-crusted lamb and a creamy herb-rich yoghurt. For a meat-free supper, swap the lamb for an extra chopped aubergine.

 4 PORTIONS PER SERVING

PREP 10 MINS
COOK 35 MINS
SERVES 4

250g diced lamb leg steak

1 aubergine, cut into 2–3cm cubes

300g natural or coconut milk yoghurt

4 garlic cloves, finely chopped

2 tbsp freshly grated ginger

a few pinches of chilli flakes

2 tbsp garam marsala

a gloss of oil (coconut, olive or ghee)

2 onions, finely diced

3 bay leaves

1 tsp fennel seeds

½ tsp ground cinnamon

400g tin of chopped tomatoes

800g tinned chickpeas

400ml water

a large handful of fresh coriander and/or mint leaves, plus extra to garnish

2 tbsp tomato purée

sea salt and freshly ground black pepper

Preheat the grill to high or oven to 220°C/Gas 7. Set a grill pan or roasting tray on the top shelf to heat up.

Tumble the lamb and aubergine into a bowl with 100g of the yoghurt, half the garlic and ginger, a pinch of chilli flakes and 1 tablespoon garam marsala. Mix well. Set aside to marinate.

Heat a large saucepan. Add a gloss of oil. Swirl in your onion. Season with salt and pepper. Cook over a medium-low heat until tender and glossy, about 5 minutes.

Swirl the bay leaves in with the onions. Add the remaining garlic, ginger and spices. Cook for a minute. Add the tomatoes. Increase the heat. Let them bubble up and reduce down a little.

Fold the chickpeas through. Pour in the water. Let them cook over a medium-low heat while you cook your skewers.

Thread the lamb and aubergine onto skewers, alternating the two. Place the skewers on the preheated pan. Grill for 10 minutes on each side.

Make a herb yoghurt by simply blending the remaining yoghurt with the herbs and a pinch of salt. (No blender? Just finely chop the herbs and fold them through the yoghurt.)

Swirl the tomato purée into the curry. Give it a taste. Adjust seasoning, as needed.

Garnish the curry with fresh herbs and little matchsticks of fresh ginger, if you like. Serve with the skewers and the yoghurt.

> **HOMEMADE GARAM MASALA**
> Toast 3 tbsp coriander seeds with 1 tbsp cumin seeds, 1 tbsp black peppercorns and 1 tsp cloves until fragrant. Grind with 1½ tsp ground ginger, seeds from 8 cardamom pods, 1 tsp ground cinnamon and 4 dried bay leaves. Cool. Store in a lidded jam jar for up to 6 months.

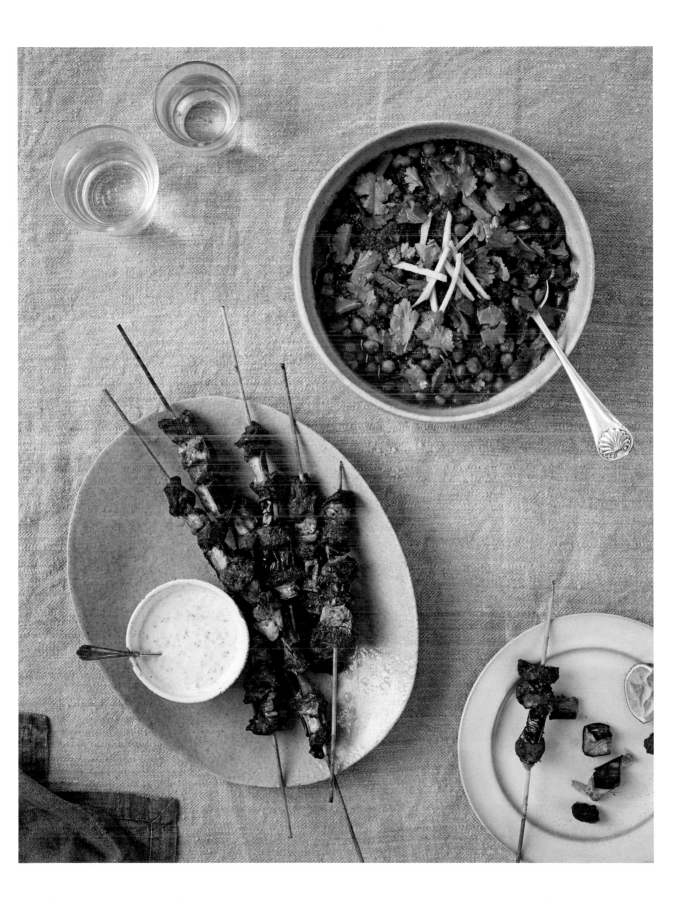

MUSHROOM PASANDA

Poet Philip Cowell introduced me to this wonderful dish. Philip and I work together at the veg box company, Abel & Cole. He had it in a restaurant, told me about it, gave me a recipe and I made up my own version using accessible ingredients. I love the wine in this dish – it gives the curry a little French twist.

 3.5 PORTIONS PER SERVING

PREP 10 MINS
COOK 30 MINS
SERVES 4

a gloss of oil (olive or coconut or ghee)

2 onions, finely chopped

600g brown, chestnut or wild mushrooms, thinly sliced or torn

1 tbsp freshly grated ginger

2 garlic cloves, finely chopped

1 tbsp curry powder

2 tsp ground turmeric

½ tsp ground cloves

¼ tsp ground cinnamon

a pinch of chilli powder (to taste)

250ml glass of white wine

600ml coconut milk

2 tbsp tomato purée

TO SERVE

a swirl of natural or Greek yoghurt (optional)

a handful of almonds, sliced and toasted (optional)

a handful of fresh coriander, roughly chopped (optional)

Heat the biggest pan you've got – the wider the base, the better. Add a generous gloss of oil. Swirl in your onion. Sizzle over a medium-low heat until just starting to soften, about 5 minutes.

Tumble in half of the mushrooms. Turn the heat up to high. Cook until the mushrooms are golden, 10 minutes. Don't be tempted to add more oil. Stir every couple of minutes.

Scrape the mushroom and onion mix into a bowl. Set aside. Put your pan back on the heat.

Once the pan's hot, add another gloss of oil. Add the remaining batch of mushrooms. Cook over a medium-high heat until golden, again about 10 minutes (depends on how big your pan is – the bigger it is, the faster they'll cook).

Fold the ginger, garlic and all the spices in with the sizzling mushrooms. Mix in your first batch of mushrooms (the ones you cooked with the onions).

Pour in the wine. Let it bubble up and reduce down a little. Swirl in the coconut milk. Let it simmer for a few minutes to thicken. Mix in the tomato purée.

Taste. Adjust the seasoning. Serve warm with a swirl of yoghurt, a scattering of toasted almonds and fresh coriander. Great with naan bread or rice.

> QUICK HOMEMADE CURRY POWDER
> Just mix the following together in a jam jar: 2 tbsp ground cumin, 2 tbsp ground coriander, 1 tbsp turmeric, ½ tsp ground ginger, ½ tsp mustard seeds (optional) and a good pinch of chilli powder (to taste). If you have some, add 1 tsp ground fenugreek but it's still stunning without it.

YELLOW MELLOW SPINACH WITH CRISPY FISH

3 PORTIONS PER SERVING

PREP 10 MINS
COOK 20 MINS
SERVES 4

a gloss of oil (coconut, olive, rapeseed or ghee)

2 onions, finely chopped

3 garlic cloves, finely chopped

4 tbsp fresh, finely grated turmeric root, or 2 tbsp ground turmeric

2 tbsp freshly grated ginger

1 chilli, finely chopped (more or less, to taste)

400g spinach

400ml coconut milk

250g tomatoes

4 fillets of hake, sea bass or bream

1 lemon or lime

a handful of toasted nigella or sesame seeds, toasted (optional)

sea salt and freshly ground black pepper

Get a large frying pan hot. Gloss with oil. Add the onions and a pinch of salt. Cook over a medium-low heat until the onions are meltingly tender, about 5 minutes.

Swirl in the garlic, turmeric, ginger and chilli. Cook until just softened.

Rinse the spinach well. Roughly chop if you're using large leaf versus baby leaf spinach.

Fold the spinach through the spiced onions and cook over a medium-heat until just softened. This will only take a minute or two. Season well. Add the tomatoes and coconut milk. Let it simmer over a low heat for 5 minutes, while you cook the fish.

Get a large pan hot. Make 2–3 slashes (about 1cm deep) across the top of each of the fish fillets, cutting into the flesh. Season well on both sides.

Add a splash of oil to the hot frying pan. Gently place the fish in the pan, skin side down. Give it a good 2–3 minutes before checking. You want the skin to really crisp up. Most of the cooking happens on the skin side.

Once the skin is really golden and crisp, gently flip the fish over. Cook flesh side down for 1–2 minutes. You'll know it's done when you can see the flesh go completely white all the way up the sides.

Tumble the tomatoes into the pan with the simmering spinach. Fold through. Taste. Adjust the seasoning as needed.

Divide the coconutty spinach and tomatoes between plates. Perch the crispy-skinned fish on top.

Pulses

THE BASICS: While I reach for tinned beans when I'm in a rush, I'm trying to get in to the habit of using dried beans instead. They're better for you (some say the lining in the aluminium tins leave harmful residue) and they're cheaper. They also have a better texture.

For perfect beans, soak the night before with 1 teaspoon of bicarbonate of soda per 100g of beans. Once cooked, 100g of dried chickpeas or beans gives you the equivalent of a 400g tin of beans. After they've soaked overnight, drain the water and put them back in the pot with fresh water. Bring to the boil. Spoon off any frothy bits off the top. Lower heat. Simmer for about 1-hour or until the beans are creamy and tender.

FRENCH PUY AND GREEN BEANS WITH CHICKEN AND MUSTARD CRÈME FRAÎCHE

If you want to swap the tinned lentils for dried, cook 200g speckled or puy lentils in 400ml water or stock for 40 minutes or until all the water is absorbed.

---

 3 PORTIONS PER SERVING

PREP 10 MINS
COOK 35 MINS
MAKES 4

---

4 chicken thighs

a few glosses of olive oil

12 sprigs of fresh thyme

1 large onion, finely diced

2 carrots, finely diced

3 sticks of celery, finely diced

3 garlic cloves, finely diced

a pinch of chilli flakes

800g tinned puy or vert lentils, drained

2 tbsp balsamic vinegar

250ml water or stock

250g French beans, trimmed

200g crème fraîche

2 tbsp Dijon mustard

a large handful of fresh tarragon leaves

sea salt and black pepper

Preheat the oven to 220°C/Gas 7.

Place the chicken in a roasting tin and season well. Add a gloss of oil and tuck all but two of the thyme sprigs around the chicken. Roast for 30 minutes or until the skin is crisp and the juices run clear when you prick the fattest part of the thighs.

Heat a large pan for the lentils and add a little oil. Tumble in the onion, carrots and celery, add a hit of salt and pepper, and sizzle over a medium-low heat until tender and glossy.

Swirl in the leaves from the remaining thyme sprigs, along with the garlic and chilli flakes. Once soft and fragrant, add the lentils and balsamic vinegar. Cook for a moment. Add 200ml of the water or stock and the French beans. Simmer until the beans are tender but still bright green about 5 minutes. Top up with more water/stock if needed.

Place the crème fraîche in a serving dish and swirl in the mustard.

Scatter half the tarragon over the lentils. Pile them on your plates and top with the chicken thighs. Scatter over the remaining tarragon. Serve with the crème fraîche mustard on the side.

ON THE ROAD TO ERITREA

Inspired by my Eritrean friend, Awot, this spice-rich dal is a delicious vegan main with rice or Injera, the traditional Eritrean sourdough flatbread. For meat eaters, it pairs beautifully with pan-fried lamb cutlets. If you can't find berbere or don't have all the spices to make it, just use a few of the spices. It'll take you in the right direction.

 PORTIONS PER SERVING

PREP   10 MINS
COOK   30 MINS
MAKES 4

200g dried red lentils

700ml water

3 onions, finely diced

a few glosses of olive oil

2 garlic cloves, finely chopped

2–3 tsp berbere

1 x 400g tin of tomatoes

50g tomato purée

a pinch of dried chillies or chilli flakes, to taste

a large handful of fresh coriander and/or parsley, chopped

sea salt

Rinse the lentils, then tip into a large pan with 600ml of the water and a pinch of salt. Bring the lentils to a boil, lower the heat and simmer for 20 minutes. When they are done, remove from the heat and set aside.

While the lentils are cooking, finely dice one of the onions. Heat a frying pan, add a gloss of oil, then tumble the onions in with a pinch of salt. Lower the heat and cook until glossy and tender.

Thinly slice the remaining onions. Heat another frying pan and add a 1cm-deep puddle of oil. Swirl the onions in with a pinch of salt and cook slowly until tender, golden and a little crisp around the edges (you'll use these golden onions to finish the dish).

Once the diced onions are soft, fold in the garlic and 2 teaspoons of berbere. Swirl in the tomatoes, tomato purée and the remaining water and simmer for 10 minutes.

Add this mix to the lentils. If you want a thicker stew, drain off any excess cooking liquid before adding the tomatoes. Simmer for 10 minutes, adding a little more water to thin, if needed. Taste, and add more berbere and/or chilli, to suit.

Serve warm with the golden onions and herbs on top.

HOMEMADE BERBERE
Classic berbere includes 8 small red chillies. As much as I love chilli, this would blow my head off. You can buy berbere pre-mixed, or make your own. In a dry frying pan, toast 2 teaspoons cumin seeds, 10 whole cloves, seeds from 10 cardamom pods, ½ teaspoon black peppercorns, ¼ teaspoon whole allspice, 1 teaspoon fenugreek and ½ teaspoon coriander seeds over a medium heat until fragrant – about 2 minutes. Remove from the heat and let cool. In a spice grinder or mortar and pestle, finely grind the toasted spices. When ground to a powder, add 1 teaspoon ground ginger, ¼ teaspoon turmeric, 1 teaspoon salt, 2½ teaspoons sweet paprika and ⅛ teaspoon cinnamon. Store in a bag or jar.

ATHENIAN RISSOLES WITH PAVLOS' SAUCE

This beautifully simple Greek tomato sauce recipe came from the mother of a friend, Pavlos Konstantineas, who shared it with me last summer. Pavlos' mother uses freshly grated tomatoes instead of passata, and you could do the same, if desired. The dish as a whole makes a light, healthy storecupboard supper, or a lovely starter for a larger Greek-themed feast.

 4 PORTION
PER SERVING

PREP 10 MINS
COOK 25 MINS
SERVES 4

FOR PAVLOS' SAUCE
a gloss of olive oil

1 onion, grated

690g passata

500ml water

½ tsp ground cinnamon

1 tsp dried oregano

sea salt and freshly ground
black pepper

FOR THE ATHENIAN RISSOLES
3 x 400g tins of chickpeas

1 large onion, grated

3 garlic cloves, finely
minced

½ tsp ground cinnamon

1 tsp chilli flakes (more or
less, to taste)

zest and juice of 1 lemon

a large handful of fresh
parsley and mint leaves,
finely chopped, plus extra
for garnish

a dusting of plain white or
chickpea (gram) flour

olive oil or ghee

For the sauce, add a gloss of oil to a saucepan, then add the grated onion and a hit of salt and pepper and cook over a medium-low heat until tender. Pour in the passata and let it bubble away for 10 minutes, until nicely thickened.

In a separate pan, warm the chickpeas in their cooking juices until tender. Drain, then add the grated onions to the warm chickpeas. Toss in the garlic, cinnamon, chilli, lemon zest and a good squeeze of juice. Add a hit of salt and pepper and pulse in a blender or food processor or mash with a potato masher or fork until you have a coarse paste. Fold the herbs through.

Add the water to the tomato sauce and bring to the boil. Swirl in the cinnamon and oregano, reduce the heat to low and let it gently bubble away for 5–10 minutes while you cook your rissoles.

Shape the chickpea mix into golf-ball-sized dumplings. The mix should give you 16 rissoles, allowing 4 per person. If the mix is a little wet, dust with flour. Press to flatten the balls a little, making patties.

Heat a 1cm deep puddle of oil in a large frying pan and shallow fry the rissoles, in batches, until golden on all sides. Make sure you give the dumplings plenty of space in the pan so they can cook evenly. Spoon the finished rissoles onto a warm plate or baking dish as you finish the others.

Taste the tomato sauce and season as needed. Spoon a good puddle of the sauce into shallow bowls or plates. Top with the warm rissoles and scatter a little fresh parsley over the top.

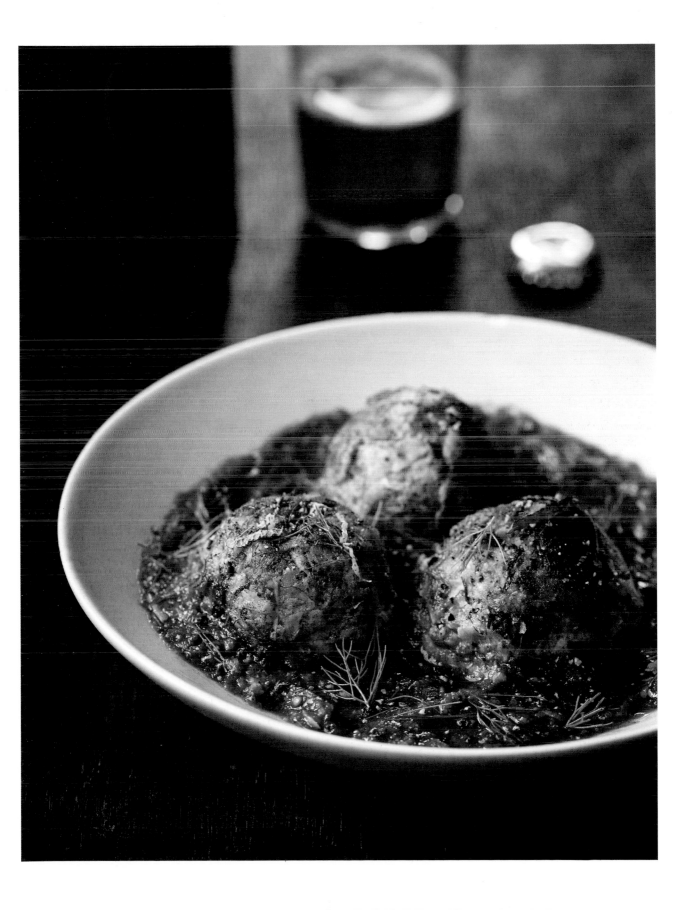

ROAST PUMPKIN AND BACON WITH CREAMY BUTTER BEAN DAL

My neighbours Joel and Paola grow pumpkins on a London farm just a few miles from my flat, and my fridge has rarely been without a pumpkin or squash since.

Crisp salty bacon is a mighty pairing for sweet, soft pumpkin. On a bed of creamy, cumin-and-cinnamon-spiced beans, it's the perfect comfort food.

 5 PORTIONS PER SERVING

PREP 5 MINS (LONGER IF USING DRIED BEANS)

COOK 45 MINS

SERVES 4

1kg pumpkin or squash

a few glosses of olive oil

8 rashers of smoked bacon, snipped into chunky lardons

4 x 400g tinned butter beans

3 garlic cloves, finely minced

1 tbsp cumin seeds

2 small cinnamon sticks or ¼ tsp ground cinnamon

a few pinches of chilli flakes

500ml veg or chicken stock

zest and juice of 1 lemon

75g rocket leaves, watercress or similar, rinsed

sea salt and freshly ground black pepper

Preheat the oven to 220°C/Gas 7. Place a large roasting tray in the oven to heat up.

Remove and discard the peel and seeds. Cut the pumpkin into 5 x 2cm chunks. Toss in a bowl with a good hit of pepper and a gloss of olive oil.

Tumble the squash into the warmed roasting tray with the bacon. Roast until the squash is tender and the bacon is golden and crisp, about 45 minutes. Remove the bacon earlier, if necessary.

Meanwhile, drain the tinned or freshly cooked beans. Heat a large pan. Add a gloss of oil. Swirl the garlic and spices through the warm oil. Add the beans and stock. Once warm, mash a few of the beans with the back of a spoon, to help thicken the broth. Add the zest and a good squeeze of juice from the lemon.

Let it bubble away over a medium-low heat until the beans are tender and have soaked up most of the stock. Top up with a little water during cooking, if necessary.

Taste the beans. Add salt, pepper and more spice, as needed. Spoon into bowls. Perch the pumpkin on the butter bean dal.

Lightly dress the rocket leaves with a little lemon juice. Pile on top. Finish with a gloss of olive oil and a pinch of chilli flakes.

COWBOY BEANS WITH MAMA'S CORNBREAD

This is a taste from my homeland. Sweet, spicy, smoky beans served with golden, sweetcorn-studded cornbread. Delicious with fresh, late-summer sweetcorn, or use frozen or tinned when corn is out of season.

PORTIONS PER SERVING

PREP   10 MINS
COOK   35 MINS
SERVES 4

1 chipotle chilli

a gloss of oil

2 onions, finely chopped

3 garlic cloves, finely minced

1 tbsp cumin seeds

½ tsp fennel seeds

1 tbsp smoked sweet paprika

a pinch of ground cinnamon

2 roasted red peppers or 6 small piquillo peppers, deseeded and finely minced

1 tbsp maple syrup

2 x 400g tins chopped tomatoes

1 tbsp cider vinegar

3 x 400g tins of mixed beans (kidney, pinto and cannellini)

200ml water

sea salt and freshly ground pepper

a handful of fresh coriander or parsley, to serve

a dollop of crème fraiche or natural yoghurt, to serve (optional)

Soak the chipotle in a mug of boiling water for 5 minutes.

Heat a pan for the beans and add a little oil. Add the onions and a pinch of salt and pepper and cook over a medium-low heat until glossy and tender.

Finely mince the chipotle. Add half (or less for a milder heat) to the onions along with the garlic. Cook for a moment, then add the cumin and fennel. Let them crackle for a second before tipping in the paprika, cinnamon, finely minced red pepper and maple syrup. Cook until reduced to a thick and sticky mix.

Pour in the tomatoes and vinegar and let it bubble up and reduce a little. Add the beans and water and bring to the boil. Reduce the heat to medium and cook for 10–15 minutes. Taste, adjusting the seasoning and spice and adding more of the chipotle chilli to suit.

Garnish with a little coriander or parsley and a swirl of crème fraîche or similar, if you wish. Serve with your fresh-from-the-oven cornbread.

MAMA'S CORNBREAD
Preheat the oven to 220°C/Gas 7. Brush the bottom and sides of a 23cm ovenproof frying pan or baking dish with oil or melted butter. Mix 125g cornmeal, 75g plain white flour, 1 tsp baking powder, ½ tsp bicarbonate of soda, ½ tsp salt and a pinch of chilli flakes in a bowl. Fold in 150g sweetcorn kernals (fresh, frozen or tinned), 6 finely chopped spring onions (or 1 finely chopped leek) and 150g grated Cheddar (smoked Cheddar is fun here). Whisk 1 egg with 200ml milk, 4 tbsp melted butter and 1 tbsp maple syrup. Fold the wet mix into the dry until thoroughly mixed. Spoon into the prepared pan. Bake for 30–35 minutes or until golden on top and coming away from the sides of the pan. Test by inserting a skewer in the centre. If it comes out clean, it's done.

Stews

THE BASICS: The word stew makes me think of slow-cooked meat and hearty root veg, snow-capped windowsills and woolly jumpers. I've never really thought of stews as speedy or summery, but once you step back and appreciate what a stew really is – ingredients cooked and served in a broth – a delicious range of edible opportunities opens up.

I've played around with a range of different stews in this section, tucking in a classic, hearty root veg mix, as well as visiting other cultures to give a taste of what the global map of stews can offer. Spices and herbs are your passports to this new world of stew-making. The swirl of harissa is what steers the Tunisian stew to North Africa; but swap the harissa for Mexican flavours and in an instant you've taken your stew to a whole new continent.

Make a beautiful broth. Add some things to it. In a nutshell, that's how you make a stew.

GREEK PENICILLIN

The perfect remedy when you're feeling feverish and achy. This dish is based on the traditional Greek soup avgolemono, but with a bundle of seasonal greens in the mix (an idea inspired by my colleague Gary Congress). If you're vegetarian, use veg stock and skip the chicken – there's enough goodness in there with the eggs and greens.

(2) PORTIONS PER SERVING

PREP 10 MINS
COOK 30 MINS
SERVES 4

½ mug of brown basmati rice

1 mug of water

1 litre chicken or veg stock

200g leftover roast chicken, shredded

5 garlic cloves, finely minced

500g seasonal greens•, cut into bite-sized pieces

2 leeks or 8–10 spring onions, cleaned and sliced

2 lemons

2 eggs

a handful of fresh roughly chopped parsley (optional)

sea salt and freshly ground black pepper

Heat a lidded pan and add the rice and a pinch of salt. Toast for a moment, then pour in the water. Pop the lid on and cook for 20 minutes, or until the rice has guzzled up all the water. Remove from the heat, lid still on, and leave to steam for 5 minutes.

Warm the stock in a large pan. Add the chicken and garlic. Once the chicken is warmed through, cram the greens and leeks or spring onions into the pan so they're fully immersed in the stock. Top up with water or more stock, if needed.

Grate the zest of both lemons into the soup. Squeeze and measure 100ml lemon juice into a mug or bowl and add the eggs. Whisk, and spoon a few ladles of the stock into the lemon/egg mix to gently warm it before slowly pouring it into the soup, stirring the whole time.

Fold the rice into the soup with a good hit of pepper. Taste. Tweak the seasoning and/or add more lemon, as needed. Divide between bowls and finish with the fresh parsley, if desired.

 SEASONAL VEG OPTIONS
Winter: broccoli, kale, shredded cabbage, mustard greens.
Spring: spring greens, nettles, wild garlic, watercress, asparagus.
Summer: broccoli, spinach, broad beans, peas, diced courgettes, fresh basil, fresh chives.
Autumn: rocket, cavolo nero, fennel.

WARMING TUNISIAN STEW WITH SMOKED FISH

This is a really simple, beautiful stew, perfect for tumbling in a heap of seasonal greens. I added the fish because I was given a smoked plaice by the most incredible fishmonger at my local food market. I perched it on top of the stew towards the end of cooking and it was a stunning addition. The dish easily stands on its own, however, so if you're vegetarian or vegan, simply leave out the fish.

 PORTIONS PER SERVING

PREP 10 MINS (LONGER IF USING DRIED BEANS)
COOK 25 MINS
SERVES 4

- a few splashes of olive oil, rapeseed oil or ghee
- 2 onions, finely chopped
- 3 garlic cloves, finely chopped
- 1 tbsp cumin seeds
- 2 tbsp tomato purée
- ½–1 tbsp harissa (more or less, to taste)
- 800g tinned chickpeas
- zest and juice of 1 lemon
- 2 litres veg, chicken or fish stock
- 75g broken spaghetti or vermicelli rice noodles
- 200–300g smoked white fish (optional)
- 4 handfuls of seasonal greens (kale, spinach, chard, wild garlic, nettles), roughly chopped
- fresh parsley, to garnish (optional)
- sea salt and freshly ground black pepper

Heat a large lidded pan and add a little oil. Sizzle the onions over a medium-low heat until tender and glossy. Swirl in a good hit of salt and pepper, then fold the garlic and cumin through. Cook for a moment before adding the tomato paste.

Add the harissa to the pan, starting with a little if you're unsure of the heat. Tumble in the chickpeas with the lemon zest and add a good squeeze of lemon juice. Top the stew up with the stock, bring to the boil, then reduce the heat to a simmer and fold the noodles in.

If adding fish, perch it on top of the stew, pop a lid on and leave it to steam for 5–10 minutes, or until the fish is cooked through. To test, pierce the fattest part of the fish: if the flesh flakes away effortlessly right the way through, it's done. Remove the fish from the stew with a slotted spoon and pull the flesh away from the skin and bones, if necessary, trying to keep it in big chunks.

Fold the greens through the stew and cook until just wilted. Taste, and adjust the seasoning, adding more lemon or harissa, to suit.

Add the flesh from the fish to the pot, or divide between bowls and perch the fish on top, garnished with a little parsley. Delicious with hunks of buttered bread.

SUMMER GARDEN POTAGE WITH BOILED EGGS

I first made this medieval-inspired dish for a lunch date with a gardener called Rose, who supplies gluts of orchard fruits and herbs to our local market stall, Patchwork Farm. The idea behind Patchwork is to encourage urban food growing and to increase the amount of local food available. Rose is always giving us beautiful things for our stall and never asks for anything in return; the least I could do was bring her lunch when I came to collect her bounty.

The veg listed in the ingredients list is just a guide, feel free to swap and change any of them for what you've got in your garden or fridge.

3 PORTIONS
PER SERVING

PREP   10 MINS
COOK   15 MINS
SERVES 4

4 duck or hens' eggs

200g fennel, roughly cut into 2cm pieces

200g fresh asparagus (if it's in season), cut into 3cm hunks, or finely diced courgettes

200g spring onions and/or wet or wild garlic, sliced

200g shelled broad beans (fresh or frozen). I also like to remove the little white coat on each bean – it's a hassle but worth it.

200g podded garden peas (fresh or frozen)

a gloss of olive oil

zest and juice of 1 lemon

a good pinch of saffron

500ml veg or chicken stock, warmed

a large handful of fresh herbs, roughly chopped

sea salt and freshly ground black pepper

Heat a pan of water and once it's boiling, add the eggs. For soft-boiled hens' eggs, gently boil for 5 minutes; for soft boiled duck eggs, boil for 8 minutes. For hard-boiled hens' eggs, boil for 8 minutes; for hard-boiled duck eggs, boil for 10 minutes. Remove the eggs from the water when boiled to your liking, rinse under cold water and set aside.

Separate the veg into piles of firm (fennel), moderately firm (asparagus, spring onions, broad beans, fresh peas, wet garlic) and delicate (thawed frozen peas, wild garlic, spinach or foraged greens).

Heat a large pan and add a gloss of oil. Add the firmer veg first with a good pinch of salt and pepper. Sizzle until just softened, then add the moderately firm veg. Again, cook until the veg starts to become tender. Add the lemon zest and squeeze in a good hit of juice. Fold the pinch of saffron through and add the stock. Once warmed through, add the delicate veg, then simmer until everything is warm and the saffron's golden hue starts to shine through. Taste, and add more seasoning, lemon and saffron, to suit.

Divide the stew between your plates and scatter a good handful of herbs over the top of each one. If you're toting the soup to a picnic or to a friend's, add the herbs just before serving as they'll lose their vibrancy if you add them to the warm soup too long before eating.

Peel the eggs and serve on the side, or halve them and perch them in the centre of your bowls, scattering some of the herbs, salt and pepper on top. Alternatively, squish the eggs between slices of generously buttered bread with a mound of herbs, salt and pepper.

The more herbs you can throw in, the merrier. I like dill, tarragon, chervil, chives, sorrel and mint. The flavour explosion this combo offers is incredible, but even just one of these herbs or some parsley, coriander or basil will do the trick.

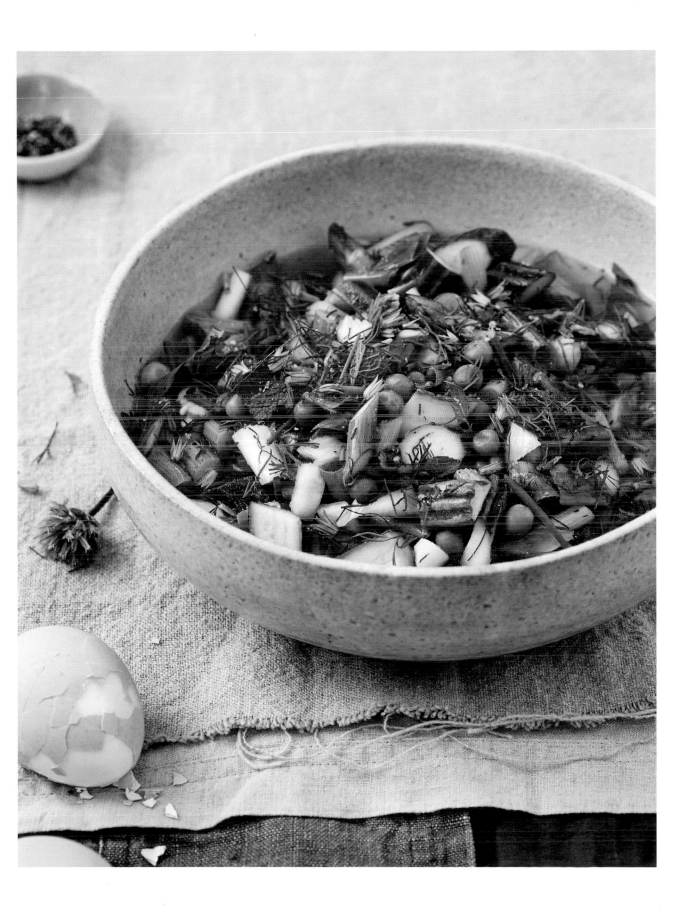

ROBBIE'S LUMBERJACK STEW

This was one of the first things my husband ever made for me, when I was pregnant with our son and certainly had the appetite of a lumberjack. This beautiful stew packs in the veg and is the perfect dish to tumble your winter root into. Avoid beetroot, though, unless you fancy a pink stew. If you have leftover beef or lamb, swirl it through when you marry the roots with the rich beer stock.

3 PORTIONS
PER SERVING

PREP 10 MINS
COOK 35 MINS
SERVES 4

1 litre veg or meat stock

750g mixed root veg
(turnips, swede, parsnips,
carrots, celeriac), peeled
and cut into 3cm hunks

500g potatoes, peeled and
cut into 3cm hunks

a gloss of olive oil

2 large onions, finely
chopped

4 garlic cloves, finely
chopped

3 sticks of celery, finely
diced

4 bay leaves, lightly torn

2 tsp finely chopped
fresh rosemary and/or
thyme leaves

1 cinnamon stick or 2 star
anise (optional)

5 tbsp tomato purée •

2 tbsp Worcestershire sauce

2 tbsp mustard

500ml dark beer (or use
more stock)

a large handful of fresh
parsley, chopped

sea salt and freshly ground
black pepper

Put the stock in a large saucepan and bring to the boil. Gently tumble the root veg and potatoes into the hot stock. Cook over a medium heat for 25 minutes, or until tender.

Heat another large pan and add a gloss of oil. Tip the onions into the pan and cook until tender. Swirl in the garlic, celery, bay, rosemary or thyme and cinnamon or star anise. Once fragrant, add the tomato purée, Worcestershire sauce, mustard and honey or maple syrup. Cook down for a moment until thick and sticky, but not beyond this so do keep an eye on it.

Pour in the beer and let it bubble up then reduce down. Swirl this rich mix into the pan with the simmering roots and stock. Let it bubble away for 10 minutes. Taste, then fine tune the flavours, adding more Worcestershire sauce, mustard and seasoning as needed. Finish with a scattering of fresh parsley.

> • *If you've got a glut of fresh tomatoes and a little extra time, finely dice 350g tomatoes (any kind). Add at the end of step 2, before adding the beer. This will add an extra portion of veg to each serving.*

Grains

THE BASICS: As with rice, the humble mug is your friend when it comes to measuring grains. The general rule of thumb is 1 mug of grains to 2 mugs of water. This amount serves 4 nicely; for 2, just halve the quantities. This method works for pretty much all grains. The exceptions are noted below.

QUINOA: I've tried to grow this one without success, but it is possible. The quinoa grains have quite a sticky (some say soapy) residue on them, so it's best to give your quinoa a good rinse before cooking. Once the water has run clear, drain, then toast the quinoa in a dry frying pan for a second before adding the water. Pop a lid on and cook over a low heat for 20 minutes, or until all the water is absorbed. Let it steam for a further 5 minutes.

BULGAR WHEAT: I never rinse this one. I just heat a large lidded pan, add the grains with a pinch of salt and toast for a moment. Then fold in a drizzle of oil, add water and pop a lid on. Cook over a low heat for 12 minutes, or until all the water is absorbed.

FREEKEH: This grain breaks the rules. I find I get the best results when I cook it like pasta. Get a pan of boiling water on the go, add the grains and boil for 15 minutes. Test to see if the grains are tender. If they are, drain the water off, leaving the grains in your sieve for a moment to allow any excess water to evaporate.

COUSCOUS: The easiest and fastest of the lot. Pour your couscous and a pinch of salt into a dish or pan with a lid. Fold in a gloss of oil, add boiling water (1 part grains to 2 parts water) and leave it to sit for 10 minutes. All the water should be absorbed in this time. Fluff up with a fork before adding your bits and bobs.

The following recipes are launch pads for other ideas. I like to add as much veg as there are grains. A nice dressing glossed over or gently mixed through is also brilliant for adding flavour and substance and for binding everything together.

Herbs and spices are brilliant for making the dish sing, while texture, in the form of crunchy nuts, seeds or crispy onions, is the icing on the cake. Soft, creamy dollops of cheese or shreds of leftover meat are further delicious additions that make for a memorable and substantial dish.

HONEYED PARSNIP QUINOA WITH CHILLI, CARDAMOM AND ORANGE

I love marrying hearty winter food with exotic, warm flavours. It works so well here. As with pretty much every dish in the book, there are lots of twists and turns you can add to make it your own.

 PORTIONS PER SERVING

PREP 10 MINS
COOK 30 MINS
SERVES 4

1kg parsnips, peeled and cut into 4cm long batons

1 large onion, thinly sliced

a pinch of chilli powder

a few glosses of olive or rapeseed oil, plus 4 tbsp for the dressing

200g quinoa

500ml water

3 oranges

1 tbsp runny honey

4 cardamom pods, seeds finely ground

a large handful of fresh parsley, finely chopped

a large handful almonds, toasted

sea salt and freshly ground black pepper

Preheat the oven to 220°C/Gas 7. Place a large roasting or baking tray on the top shelf of the oven to warm up.

Toss the parsnips and onion in a bowl with a little salt, pepper and chilli powder. Gloss with just enough oil to lightly coat. Tumble onto the warmed tray and roast for about 25–30 minutes, or until golden and tender.

Meanwhile, rinse your quinoa in a fine mesh sieve. Heat a lidded pan and toast the rinsed grains for a moment. Swirl in a pinch of salt and a drop of oil. Pour in the water, pop a lid on, lower the heat and let it cook for 20 minutes, or until all the water is fully absorbed. Remove from the heat, lid still on, and leave to steam for a further 5 minutes. Drain any excess water.

Halve one of the oranges. Squeeze out 8 tablespoons of juice into a clean, lidded jam jar. Mix with the 4 tablespoons of olive oil, a pinch of salt, the honey and ground cardamom. Shake or whisk until fully emulsified. Taste and adjust the seasoning and the orange/oil/honey ratio to your liking.

Once the parsnips are nearly done, pour a little dressing over them, just enough to lightly coat, and pop them back in the oven for a couple of minutes, allowing the dressing to turn to a sticky glaze.

Cut the remaining oranges into 1cm-thick rounds – whip the peel off the rounds. Mix them through the quinoa, along with the chopped parsley and the remaining dressing. Tuck the roasted parsnips in to the mix, once cooked. Scatter the toasted almonds over the top. Serve warm or cold.

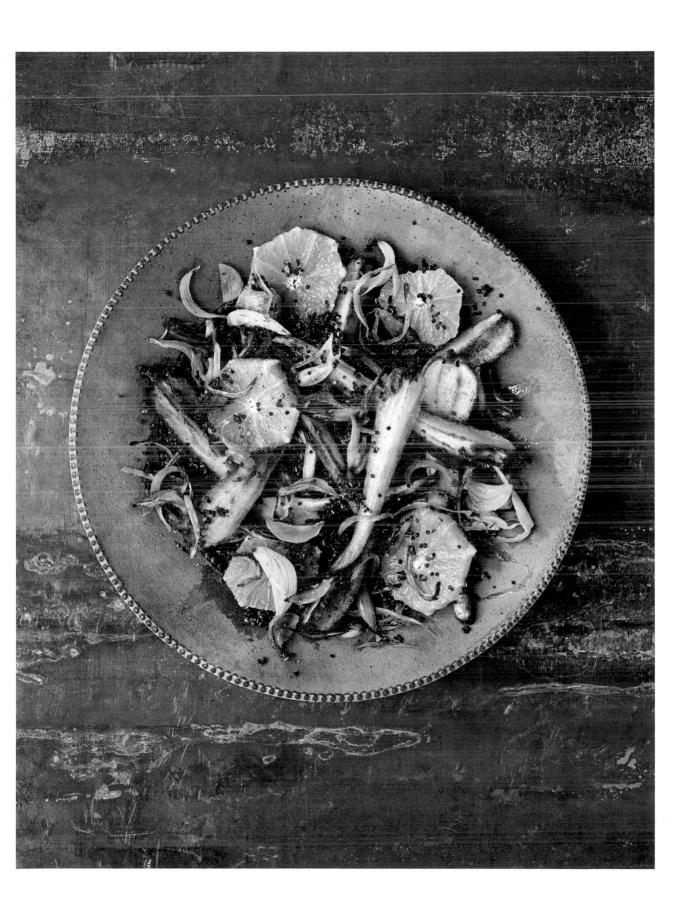

TOASTED WALNUT QUINOA WITH GREENS, MUSTARD AND CURED MEAT

This light supper packs in the nutrients and is a brilliant on-the-go dish. It's something I crave often. Unless I'm famished, I find this dish satisfying enough on its own, but to add more bulk perch a poached egg on top.

 PORTIONS PER SERVING

1.5

PREP 5 MINS
COOK 25 MINS
SERVES 4

1 mug of quinoa (I love using red quinoa purely for aesthetic purposes, but use what you've got)

2 garlic cloves, finely minced

2 mugs of water

1 tbsp Dijon mustard

2 tbsp balsamic or red wine vinegar

75ml olive oil

400g seasonal greens, cleaned and roughly chopped

12–16 wafer-thin slices of cured meat, such as Parma ham or bressaola

a handful of walnuts, toasted

sea salt and freshly ground black pepper

Rinse the quinoa well. Heat a lidded pan and add the quinoa to the hot pan with the garlic, a pinch of salt and pepper and the water. Pop a lid on, simmer for 20 minutes, or until the quinoa is tender and all the water is absorbed.

Pour the mustard, vinegar and oil into a clean, lidded jam jar. Pop a lid on and shake until creamy and beautifully mixed.

As soon as the quinoa's done, remove from the heat and pile the greens on top. Put the lid back on and let the greens steam for a moment, until just tender but still a bright, glossy green.

Swirl the greens through the quinoa, scatter over a pinch of pepper and divide between plates. Drizzle the dressing over, serving any extra on the side. Drape the cured meat on top, scatter the nuts over and tuck in.

● *I've used all sorts of greens in this dish: chard, beetroot leaves, wild garlic, spinach, kale and broccoli leaves.*

CARROT PILAF WITH AVOCADO, PISTACHIO AND SAFFRON CRÈME FRAÎCHE

This dish is the happy marriage of a trip to an Isle of Wight farm shop and the discovery of a thirteenth-century recipe from Baghdad. To my surprise, this rural island farm shop sold freekeh and a host of Middle Eastern spices alongside their local produce, but if you can't find freekeh, swap for bulgar wheat or quinoa.

 4.5 PORTIONS
PER SERVING

PREP   10 MINS
COOK   45 MINS
SERVES 4

750g carrots (go for a mix of colourful summer bunched carrots)

400g shallots or onions, thinly sliced

a few glosses of olive oil

zest and juice of 1 lemon

a good pinch of saffron

1 tbsp boiling water

200g freekeh

2 garlic cloves, finely minced

2 tsp ground cinnamon

2 tsp ground cumin or cumin seeds

200g crème fraîche

a large handful of fresh coriander, parsley and/or mint, chopped

a small handful of leafy green carrot tops (if available), chopped

2 ripe avocados, peeled and sliced

100g pistachios, shelled and lightly crushed

sea salt and freshly ground black pepper

Preheat the oven to 220°C/Gas 7. Place a large roasting tray in the oven to heat up.

Scrub the carrots clean and halve or quarter them lengthways. Toss the carrots and shallots or onions in a bowl with a pinch of salt, pepper, a gloss of oil and the grated lemon zest and a good squeeze of juice. Tumble into the warmed roasting dish. Cook for 45 minutes or until tender and golden around the edges.

Meanwhile, drop the saffron into a small dish or tea cup. Pour the boiling water over, give it a little stir and set aside to infuse.

Place the freekeh in a saucepan with 1 litre of water and a pinch of salt. Bring to the boil, then reduce the heat and simmer for 15 minutes. Drain, and toss with the minced garlic cloves and a gloss of oil.

As soon as your carrots and shallots are done, fold the cinnamon and cumin through.

Mix the saffron and the soaking liquid through the crème fraîche and set aside.

Tumble the freekeh into a dish with the carrots and shallots and fold everything together. Taste, and adjust the seasoning, if needed. Plate up the pilaf, scattering most of the herbs over the top.

Dot the avocados into the mix. Add a hit of lemon juice and a gloss of olive oil, followed by the remaining herbs and the pistachios. Drizzle the saffron crème fraîche over the top or serve dolloped on the side.

LEMON DILL BULGAR WHEAT WITH FRIED COURGETTES AND GOAT'S CURD

A beautiful summery dish. If you're dairy free, swap the goat's curd for toasted almonds. For gluten free diets, swap the bulgar wheat for quinoa.

 2.5 PORTIONS
PER SERVING

PREP   10 MINS
COOK   25 MINS
SERVES 4

225g bulgar wheat

a few splashes of olive or rapeseed oil

750ml water or stock

4 garlic cloves, crushed flat and papery skin removed

4 courgettes (about 750g), sliced into thin rounds

a pinch of chilli powder

zest and juice of 1 lemon

2 large handfuls of fresh dill, roughly chopped

a large handful of pistachios, toasted

200g goat's curd (or a similar cheese or Greek yoghurt)

a dusting of sumac (optional)

sea salt and freshly ground black pepper

Heat a lidded pan, add the bulgar wheat and toast for a moment. Swirl in a pinch of salt, pepper and a drop of oil, then pour in the water or stock and put the lid on. Lower the heat and cook for 12 minutes, or until all the water is absorbed. Remove from the heat, lid still on, and leave to steam for a further 5–10 minutes.

Heat a large frying pan and add a gloss of oil. Fry the garlic cloves over a medium heat until they're starting to colour. Spoon out and toss in with the grains.

Season the courgette rounds well with salt, pepper and a little chilli powder.

Cook the courgettes in the garlicky oil, in batches so you can keep them in a single layer, until they're nice and golden on each side. Taste, and adjust the seasoning, as needed.

Add the lemon zest and juice to the grains – taste as you add it; if your lemons are extra juicy, you may not need all the juice. Fold a generous amount of herbs through; you want the grains to be green and fragrant.

Scatter the courgettes and nuts over the grains, gently mixing them through. Finish with dollops or crumbles of cheese and a dusting of sumac or a little more black pepper.

Variation: use the bulgar wheat as a base for these trios:

– Roasted carrots, basil, pine nuts.
– Garden peas, mint, edible flowers.
– Aubergines rubbed with harissa, parsley, pomegranate seeds.
– Cherry tomatoes, chives, poppy seeds.
– Avocado, coriander leaves, sunflower and pumpkin seeds.

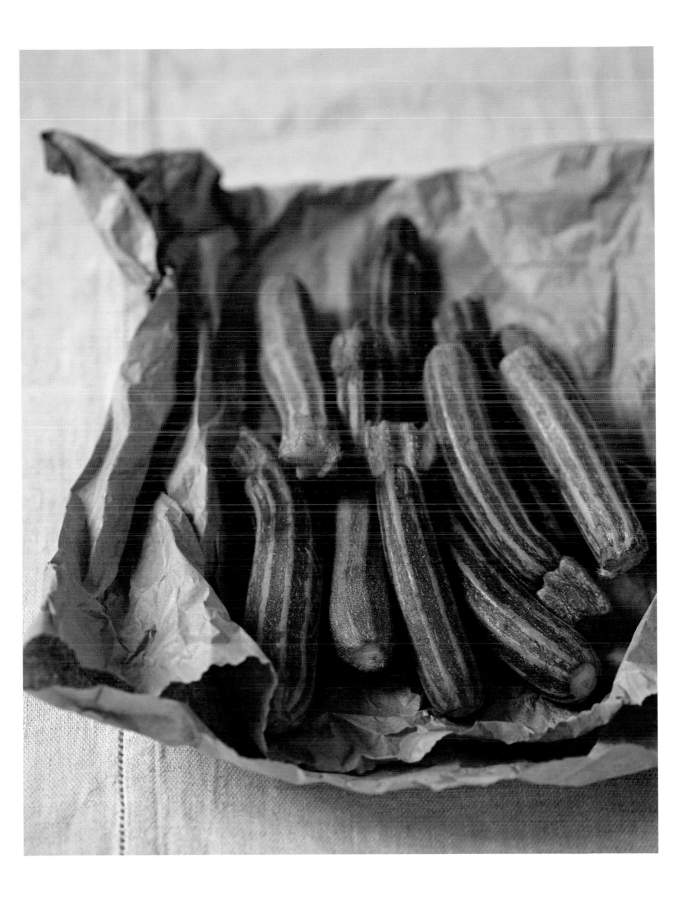

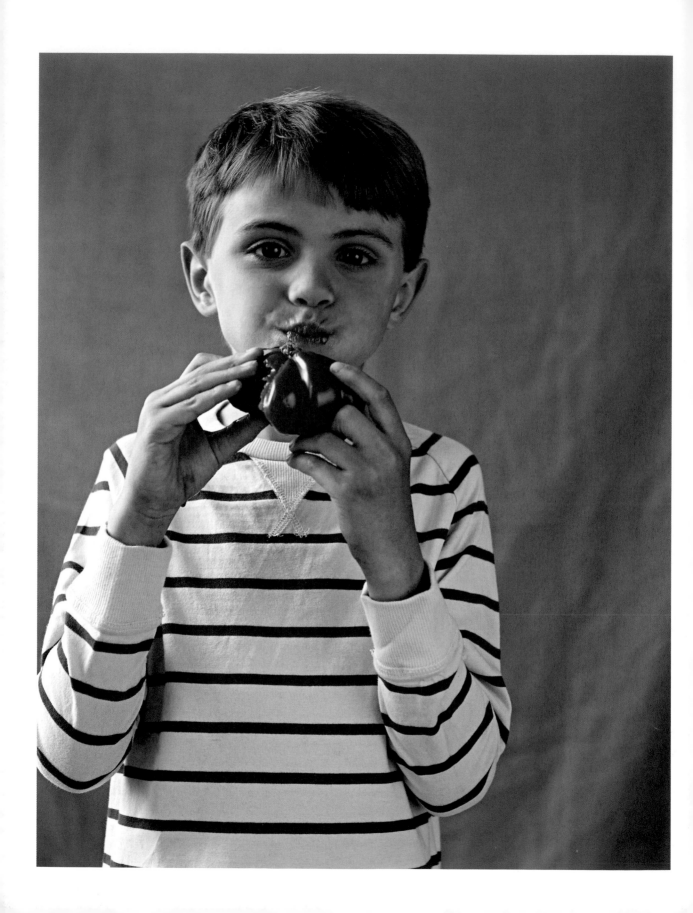

BITE: CHILDREN AND VEG

Children approach a plate of food as if they were hunter/gatherers in the wild. They need to sniff, touch, look and effectively play with their food to feel confident that it is indeed edible. If you've ever been foraging, you can probably relate to this. You don't just go up to a shrub and start eating the berries. You have to examine them first. Engaging children with food through play and sitting down to eat dinner with them are to key ways to help the get over these barriers. Playing with fruit and veg, using some of the ideas below, makes food fun and fascinating, and less of a fret or fear. And come meal time, if you are there eating alongside your children, showing them that the food is indeed safe to eat, and delicious, then it's pretty likely that they'll want to get stuck in.

Shell and schuck: Get them to help you shell peas and broad beans, and shuck sweetcorn, peeling the outer greens and silky threads off. It's quite useful when they get the knack, and it's a great way to get their hands on veg without being pressured to eat it.

Spice it up: Spices are also a great way of introducing little ones to the magic of the kitchen. Let them help you grind spices and make spice blends. This is especially helpful if you're trying to get them interested in curry. My son and I also play a blindfold game where we smell, taste and touch different spices (as well as fruits and vegetables), guessing what they are simply by smelling, tasting or touching them.

Paint by veg: Using the colours produced by fruit and veg is brilliant fun. When my son was edging towards age one, we foraged for blackberries and used them to splat on paper to make a painting (of sorts). We've also had fun printing with beetroot and we've made paintbrushes with the silky threads hidden beneath the greens of late summer sweetcorn.

One potato, two potato: This is one of the best things you can do as it really helps with their math skills: get them into the kitchen and let them help you count out (one potato, two potato, three potato, four . . .), weigh and measure the ingredients. If you're working from a recipe, get them to help you read it too. Even if they're too young to read on their own, it will really help them cross that bridge once they come to it.

Funny face: My friend Tania did this when my son came over and he's always raving about it. Lay out a selection of cut or whole fruits on a table. Give each child a plate and invite them to invent a face for a character. Then ask them to tell a story about their character. If there are several children, see if they can incorporate the other characters in their story.

FEAST

Japanese Feast

My husband always asks, 'If you could only ever eat one type of food for the rest of your life, which would it be?' It's a tricky one, but I think Japanese tops the list. I love its beautiful dance of flavours and textures; the interplay of sweet and salty, fresh and rich.

When I was writing for *Waitrose Food Illustrated,* I hosted an airline food taste test with a panel of chefs and food writers. The Japanese even get airline food right. The trays from Nippon Airlines were so interactive and engaging, with little pots and sachets of sauces for dipping: spicy pyramids of wasabi for your sushi; sweet and sour wisps of ginger; crunchy little pickles. Japanese food really does invite you to dive in. It's healthy and light, and though the Japanese love their meat and fish, seasonal vegetables and fruit play a central role.

JAPANESE FEAST MENU

~

English Edamame with Lemon Sea Salt

*

Spiced Alfalfa, Avocado and Cashew Sushi

*

Saucy Miso Spinach with Toasted Sesame

Ginger Chicken and Spring Onion Yakitori Skewers

*

Wild Mushroom Hot Pot

[THE FULL MENU OFFERS EACH DINER 6 PORTIONS]

SPICED ALFALFA, AVOCADO AND CASHEW SUSHI

This rice-less, veg-laden roll is the easiest sushi you can make, and it's super-healthy. It's perfect with the little turnip pickles below. You could also serve with a small dish of mirin or soy sauce for dipping.

 2 PORTIONS
PER SERVING

PREP **20** MINS
COOK NIL
SERVES **6**

200g alfalfa sprouts

1 tbsp freshly grated ginger

a few shakes of soy sauce

8–10 sheets of nori seaweed

1 large or 2 small ripe
avocados

a pinch of chilli flakes
(optional)

4 tbsp cashews, toasted

Have a little dish of water at the ready for your sushi-making. You'll use this to dampen and seal the sushi rolls.

Mix the sprouts, ginger and a few shakes of soy sauce in a large bowl. Taste. Add a little more soy or ginger, to your liking.

If you've got a bamboo rolling mat, lay it on a cutting board or a firm surface. If not, no worries – just use your hands. Lay a sheet of nori on your mat or surface. Brush with water. Lay another sheet on top, so you have a double layer of seaweed.

Dip your index finger in the water. Run it along the top and bottom 1cm of the sheet. Pile a mound of the sprouts in the centre. Spread to create a 1cm thick layer, leaving a 1cm gap at the top and bottom.

Halve and stone the avocado. Remove the peel. Thinly slice. Arrange a few avocado slices in a line in the bottom third of the roll. Scatter a pinch of chilli flakes and a line of cashews beneath the avocado.

Using your mat or your fingers to help keep everything firmly tucked in, gently roll the filled nori sheet from bottom (the side nearest to you) to top. If the filling starts to spill out, just pinch it out or tuck it back in. Keep going until you've got a log-like shape. Dab extra water on the seam to seal, if needed.

With the roll seam-side down, cut it into 3–4cm-thick rolls (a serrated knife works well here). You should get around 5–6 cut rolls. Repeat until all the nori sheets and filling are used up and serve.

LITTLE TURNIP PICKLES
Quarter 250g turnips. Slice as thinly as possible. Mix the slices in a bowl with 3 strips of lemon zest and 1 tsp sea salt. Scrunch everything together with your hands for about 5 minutes. Liquid will start to come out of the turnips and the veg will start to soften. Drain off the liquid. Cover with a plate or bowl that will fit nicely on top of your pickles. Weight it down, so it helps press more liquid out of the veg. Leave to sit for 1 hour. Place the pickles in a sieve or colander and rinse well in cold water. Pile into a dish and serve with your sushi.

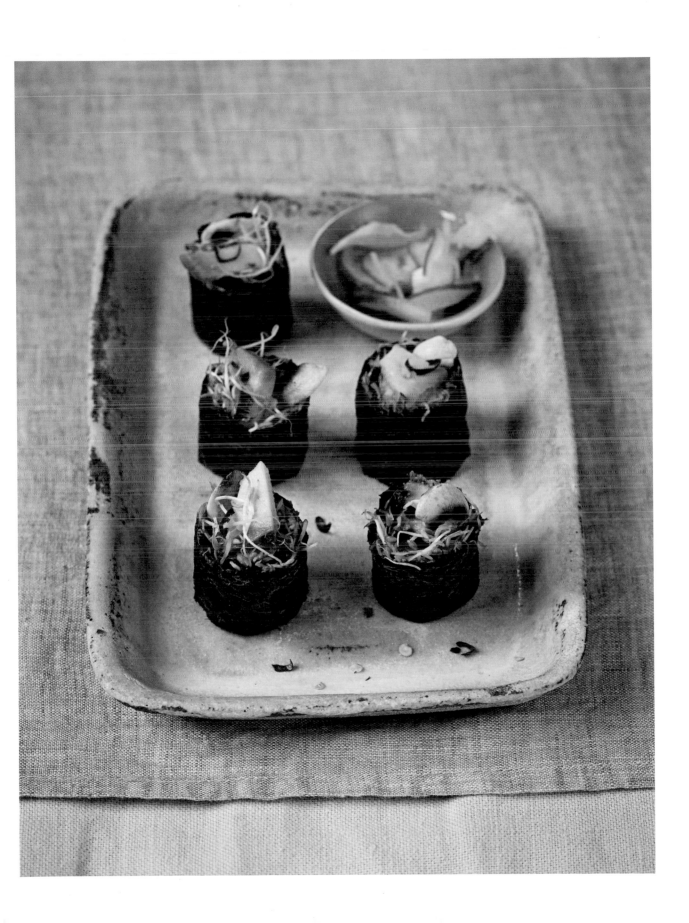

ENGLISH EDAMAME WITH LEMON SEA SALT

Sugar snap peas are one of the first gems to appear in an English summer garden. As you can eat the whole thing, skin and all, they're a great alternative to edamame.

 1 PORTION
PER PERSON

PREP   5 MINS
COOK   5 MINS
SERVES 6

500g sugar snap peas•

1 lemon

a pinch of sea salt

1 tbsp sesame seeds

Heat a large frying pan. No oil is needed. Rinse the peas and toss them in the hot pan while they still have a little water clinging to them. Sizzle until they're just tender, bright green and a little charred.

Add a grating of lemon zest, a squeeze of juice and a pinch of salt. Toss in the sesame seeds and toast for a second, then tumble everything onto a serving dish and eat hot.

> • *Garden peas still in the pod or young, tender broad beans can also be used. Eat them like edamame, tugging the beans/peas out of their pods with your teeth.*

SAUCY MISO SPINACH WITH TOASTED SESAME

 1 PORTION
PER SERVING

PREP   10 MINS
COOK   10 MINS
SERVES 6

4 tbsp sesame seeds

1 tbsp miso paste (any kind; a richer, dark miso is ideal)

1 tbsp water

1 tsp runny honey

1 tsp freshly grated ginger

500g baby or smaller, tender spinach leaves

a few chilli flakes, to garnish (optional)

Heat a large frying pan and add the sesame seeds. Lower the heat and toast gently until golden. Tip into a dish and set aside.

Whisk the miso paste, water, honey and ginger together until fairly smooth and fully mixed.

Rinse the spinach thoroughly. Return the empty frying pan to the heat. Add the spinach and gently fold it through the pan, just to wilt it. Swirl the miso mixture through until it's melting into the spinach.

Pile onto a serving dish and scatter over the toasted sesame seeds, along with a pinch of chilli flakes, if you like.

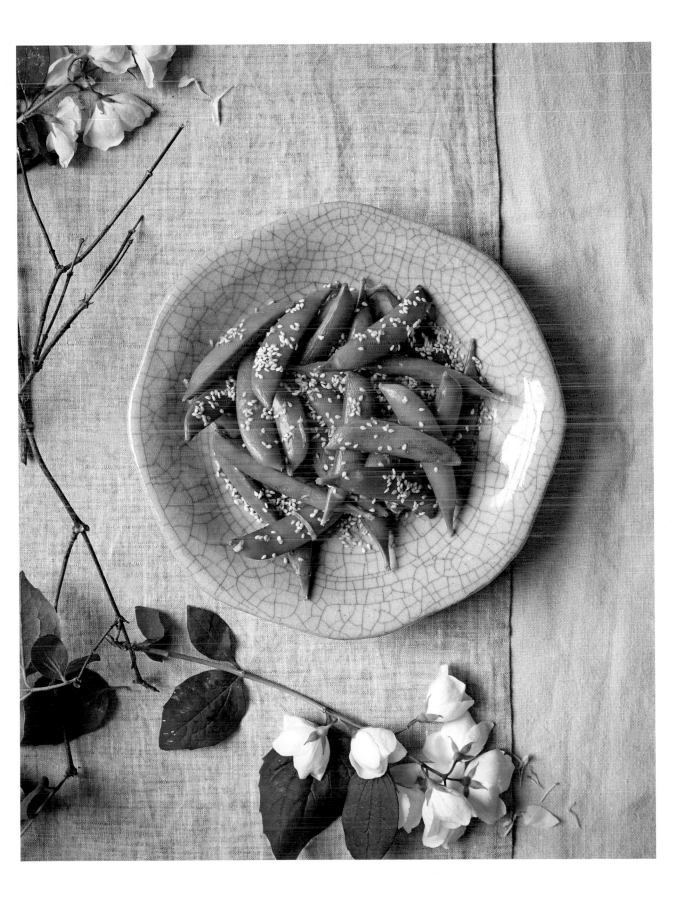

GINGER CHICKEN AND SPRING ONION YAKITORI SKEWERS

My boys love these, either paired with other Japanese dishes, as a snack, or as a simple supper with noodles and some stir-fried veg.

0.5 PORTION PER SERVING

PREP   15 MINS
COOK   15 MINS
SERVES 6

5 tbsp mirin

3 tbsp soy sauce

2 tbsp runny honey, maple syrup or sugar (or your favourite sweetener)

500g chicken (breasts, thighs or leg meat), cut into 3cm hunks

1 tbsp finely grated ginger

150g spring onions (or leeks or normal onions, if preferred)

2 tbsp sesame seeds, toasted

Preheat the grill to high or oven to 220°C/Gas 7. Place a grill pan or baking sheet in the oven to heat up.

Mix the mirin with the soy sauce and your sweetener of choice.

Tumble the diced chicken into a bowl. Pour the mirin marinade over and fold in the ginger. Leave to marinate for as long as you can – at least 15 minutes or ideally overnight.

Rinse the spring onions and trim the root ends off. Cut both the whites and greens into 3cm hunks.

Thread the marinated chicken and spring onions onto 12 skewers, alternating the two (add 3–4 hunks of onion for each 1 hunk of chicken). Save any marinade left over from the chicken.

Grill or cook the skewers on the preheated pan, on the top shelf, for 5–10 minutes on each side, or until nicely browned and cooked through. Gloss with the remaining marinade a couple of times during cooking.

Scatter the toasted sesame seeds over just before serving.

Variation: for a vegan/vegetarian option swap the chicken for parboiled or steamed hunks of squash or tofu (roughly 3cm cubes).

● *If you can't find mirin, swap for 2 tbsp soy sauce mixed with 2 tbsp water, ½ tbsp cider or rice vinegar and ½ tbsp sweetener of your choice.*

WILD MUSHROOM HOT POT

A dish that will forever linger in my memory is the crab rice hot pot served at Roka, a Japanese restaurant in London. While I've never seen their recipe, this is my nod to utterly moreish and comforting Japanese-style hot pots. Mine is far from authentic, but it's really easy to make and hits all those lovely flavour and texture notes beautifully. The portions here serve 6 as a side or 4 as a main.

 1.5 PORTIONS PER SERVING

PREP 15 MINS
COOK 30 MINS
SERVES 6

1 litre veg or chicken stock

a few glosses of olive or sesame oil

9 white onions or 12–16 spring onions, finely chopped

9 garlic cloves, finely chopped

1 red chilli, finely chopped (more or less, to taste)

4 tbsp freshly grated ginger

200g risotto rice

a few shakes of soy sauce

500g mushrooms, torn or thinly sliced•

a large handful of wild garlic or chives, roughly chopped

Pour the stock into a saucepan, place over a medium heat and bring to a gentle simmer.

Heat a second pan and add a gloss of oil and the onions. Lower the heat and cook until translucent and tender.

Mix the garlic, chilli and ginger in a bowl. Remove a good-sized pinch and set aside, then swirl the rest through the onions and cook until softened. Add the rice, mix through, toast for a moment and add a few shakes of soy sauce.

Pour a ladle of the simmering stock onto the rice. Set a timer for 20 minutes and continue to feed the stock to the rice, little by little, stirring often, until the timer goes off and the rice is tender.

While the rice cooks, sizzle the mushrooms in a frying pan with a little oil until golden. Swirl in the reserved pinch of garlic/chilli/ginger and cook for a moment. Splash in a little soy sauce to coat.

When the rice is ready, fold the mushrooms through or serve them perched on top. Stir in most of the wild garlic or chives, saving a handful to scatter over the dish just before you serve it.

> • *A wild mix of spring mushrooms is a delight in this dish, but any variety from chestnut mushrooms to shiitakes to portobellos will work. My favourite are morels, but they're not cheap. A 50/50 mix of wild and cultivated mushrooms is a happy compromise.*

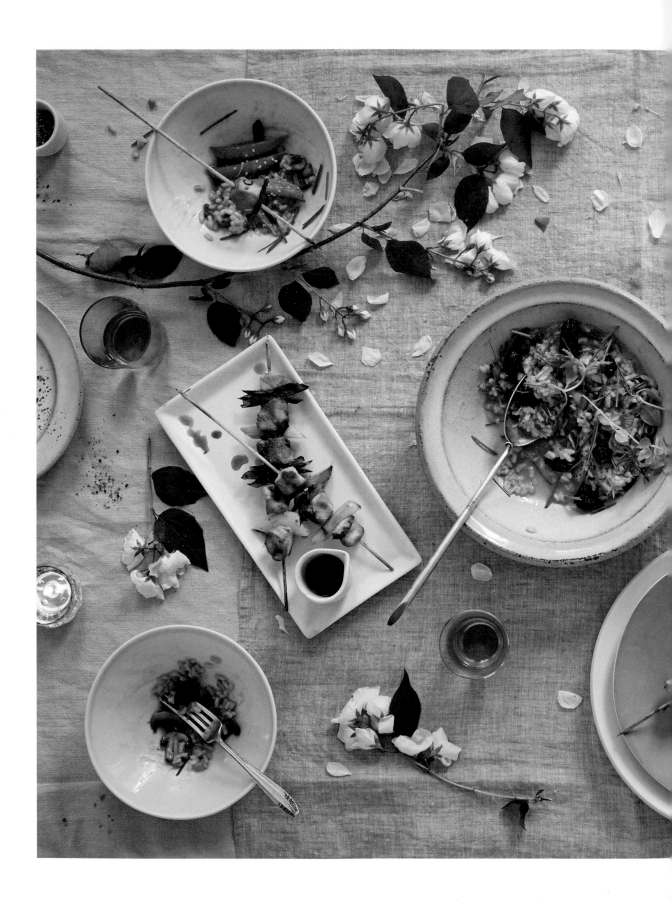

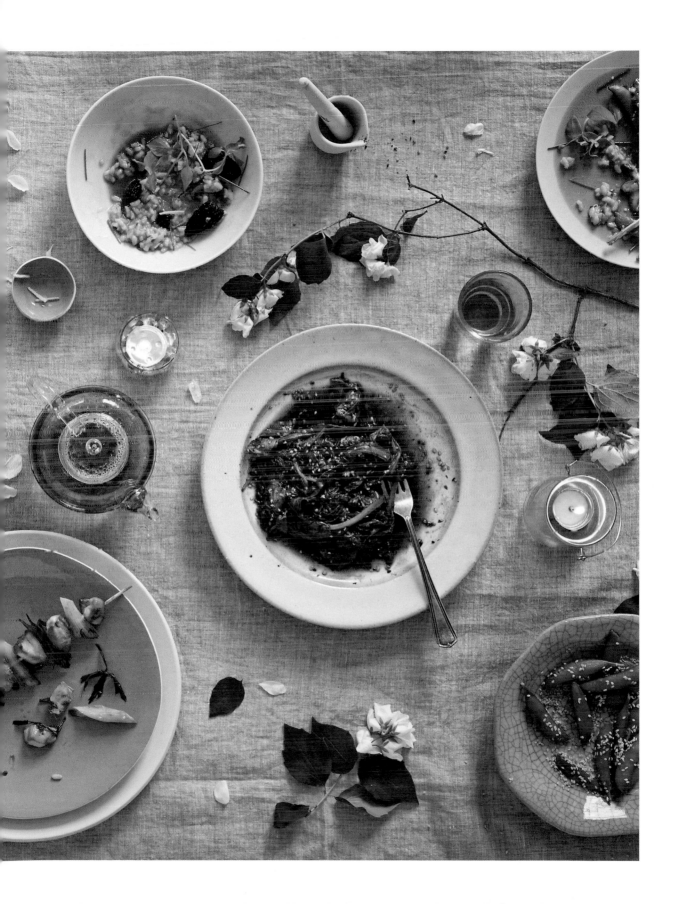

New Orleans Feast

While most people's image of Southern cooking probably veers toward big slabs of meat, grits and lots of deep-fried things, the cuisine of my childhood is rich and bountiful on the fruit and veg front; because we're talking sunny climes here, the selection is immense. One of the things I miss most about home are my granddad's watermelons and orchards of fragrant peaches. Last time I strolled around his garden, my son plucked out a spring onion the size of a leek. And the tomatoes are so bountiful my granny could hardly keep up with them, transforming them into salsas, my favourite pickle (chow-chow), or freezing them whole for later in the year.

The joy of Texas cuisine is that it is influenced from all directions. There's Mexico to the south, Louisiana to the east, and then you get some really interesting Native American flavours mixed with a drift of Californian cuisine from the west. There's also a strong Pennsylvanian Dutch influence. Many of my own favourite tastes from home have Creole roots: my momma's gumbo and black-eyed peas are great comfort foods. If you want to wash down the following feast in true Southern style, forget the beer or wine, it has a be a jug of sweet iced tea, brewed in the heat of the sun. Or if the weather's not up for brewing tes, plump for a homemade mint julep to kick things off.

NEW ORLEANS FEAST MENU

~

Corn-crusted Courgette Straws with Jivin' Chive Dip

*

Summer Veg Patch Gumbo with Chorizo and Crab

Healthy Hoppin' John

Mardi Gras Slaw with Maple Pecans

*

Inside Out Blackberry Cobbler

[THE FULL MENU OFFERS EACH DINER 5.5 PORTIONS]

CORN-CRUSTED COURGETTE STRAWS WITH JIVIN' CHIVE DIP

Not the healthiest dish in the book, but it's a traditional taste from my days in the Deep South and it's a brilliant way to get courgettes into the mouths of those who claim to loathe them.

 PORTION PER SERVING

PREP	10 MINS
COOK	20 MINS
SERVES	6

3 large courgettes

zest and juice of 2 lemons

1 mug of cornmeal or fine polenta

2 eggs, beaten

rapeseed oil, coconut oil or ghee, for shallow frying

2 pinches of cayenne pepper

200g crème fraîche

½ tsp maple syrup, agave or runny honey

2 tbsp finely chopped chives

chive flowers (if available) or extra chives, to garnish (optional)

sea salt and freshly ground black pepper

Cut the courgettes into batons, roughly 8cm long and 2cm thick. Scatter over half the lemon zest and juice of 1 lemon and dust with a good hit of salt and pepper.

Tip half the cornmeal mixture into a shallow dish or plate, then dredge the lemony courgettes through to lightly coat. Put the beaten eggs in a second shallow dish and dip each baton in the egg. Add the remaining cornmeal to the first plate and coat the egg-dipped courgette batons in the cornmeal, one at a time, to give a final coating.

Heat a large shallow frying pan until smoking hot. Add a shallow puddle of oil, about 1cm deep, then gently place the courgette batons in the hot oil, in a single layer, with a little room around each. Fry in batches until golden on all sides, turning as needed. Once cooked, dust with a little salt and a pinch of cayenne.

In a small serving bowl, mix the crème fraîche with a pinch of salt, pepper, a hint of cayenne, a grating of zest from the remaining lemon and about 2 tablespoons of lemon juice, and the maple syrup, agave or honey. Fold the chopped chives through. Taste, and adjust the seasoning, spice and sweetness to your liking.

Scatter chive flowers over the courgette straws and serve with the yoghurt dip.

SUMMER VEG PATCH GUMBO WITH CHORIZO AND CRAB

Nothing says New Orleans like a bubbling hot pot of gumbo. Most people think of Cajun food as laden with spice; in reality it's all about subtle hints of heat. To keep the dish friendly to all chilli-tolerances, you can be flexible with the amount of cayenne, especially as some brands differ hugely in strength.

PORTIONS PER SERVING

PREP 20 MINS
COOK 1 HOUR
SERVES 6

100g chorizo

olive oil or ghee

3 tbsp plain white or chickpea flour, plus extra for dusting

1 large onion, finely diced

3 sticks of celery, finely diced

1 green pepper, diced

4 garlic cloves, finely minced

3 fresh bay leaves, torn

1 tsp dried basil

1 tsp dried or fresh thyme

2 tsp sweet paprika

2 pinches of cayenne pepper

400g of chopped tomatoes

1 litre shellfish, chicken or veg stock

2 tsp cider or sherry vinegar

a good shake of chilli sauce

3 ears fresh sweetcorn, cut into 3cm thick rounds

200g fresh crab meat (100% white or a 50/50 mix)

150–200g okra, cut into 1cm rounds

zest and juice of 1 lemon

a large handful of fresh coriander and/or parsley

sea salt and ground pepper

Heat a large pan until smoking hot. If using cooking chorizo, remove the skin and break into little pieces. If using a tougher, cured chorizo, cut into 1cm cubes. Tumble the chorizo into the pot and let it sizzle for a few minutes and render out some of its fat and flavour. Spoon the chorizo out and set aside.

Add enough oil to the chorizo oil to make 3 tablespoons. Once warm, swirl in the flour and whisk constantly to form a smooth paste. Cook over a medium heat until it darkens to a milk chocolate brown; this is your roux, a classic base to a good gumbo, adding thickness and a rich underlying flavour.

Add the onion, celery and pepper to the roux. Swirl through and cook over a medium heat until tender. Fold in the garlic, bay leaves and a hit of salt and pepper. If at any stage the mix is getting too thick or dry, just add a splash of stock, but keep it relatively thick and pasty at this stage – though don't let it burn.

Mix in the basil, thyme, paprika and a pinch of cayenne pepper. Then add the chopped tomatoes and the cooked chorizo. Let them bubble up and reduce down a bit before adding the stock, vinegar and a shake of chilli sauce. Simmer for 15 minutes to infuse all the flavours. Then add the sweetcorn and crab meat.

Heat a frying pan for the okra (frying it off before adding it to the gumbo will give it a nicer texture). Season the okra with salt, pepper and a hint of cayenne pepper, and dust with just enough flour to lightly coat. Add a good gloss of oil to the pan and shallow fry the okra until golden all over. Add to your gumbo just before serving.

Finish the gumbo with a grating of lemon zest and a little juice. Taste, and adjust the seasoning, adding more cayenne or chilli sauce, to suit. You can also add a hit of Worcestershire sauce if you like, but I find it a little overpowering. Once you've fine-tuned the flavour, scatter the herbs over and serve.

HEALTHY HOPPIN' JOHN

I grew up eating Hoppin' John, though we never called it by this brilliant name. The traditional dish is a stew of black-eyed peas with bacon or ham, eaten by folks across America's Deep South on New Year's Day to bring luck for the forthcoming year. It's served with collard greens or cabbage and cornbread, both symbolic of wealth in the year ahead. On the day after New Year's Day, leftover Hoppin' John is called Skippin' Jenny, demonstrating frugality and bringing hope for an even better chance of prosperity in the New Year.

Renowned Southern cookery writer Paula Deen introduced me to his healthy twist to Hoppin' John. It is the perfect side dish for hearty gumbo.

 PORTIONS PER SERVING

PREP	5 MINS (LONGER IF USING DRIED BEANS)
COOK	25 MINS
SERVES	6

1 mug of quinoa (red or a multi-coloured quinoa, if possible)

a few glosses of olive oil

2 mugs of water

1 pepper (any colour), finely diced

2 sticks of celery, finely diced

1 tsp cumin seeds

1 tsp fresh or dried thyme leaves

400g of black-eyed peas, drained and rinsed, or 100g dried beans soaked overnight and cooked until tender

2 tsp Dijon mustard

a pinch of cayenne pepper

6 spring onions, thinly sliced

zest and juice of 1 lemon

a large handful of fresh coriander or parsley, roughly chopped

sea salt and ground pepper

Heat a lidded pan. Rinse the quinoa and add it to the hot pan with a pinch of salt and a drop of oil. Pour in the water, lower the heat and pop the lid on. Cook for 20 minutes, or until the quinoa is tender and all the water is absorbed.

Place a frying pan over a high heat and add a gloss of oil. Tumble in the pepper and celery with a pinch of salt and pepper. Sizzle over a medium heat until just tender. Sprinkle in the cumin and thyme and mix everything together.

Add the drained beans to the pepper and celery. Swirl in the mustard and cayenne, along with a trickle of water, just enough to moisten. Remove the pan from the heat and fold the spiced beans, spring onions, lemon zest and a good squeeze of juice through the quinoa when it's ready. Finish with the herbs.

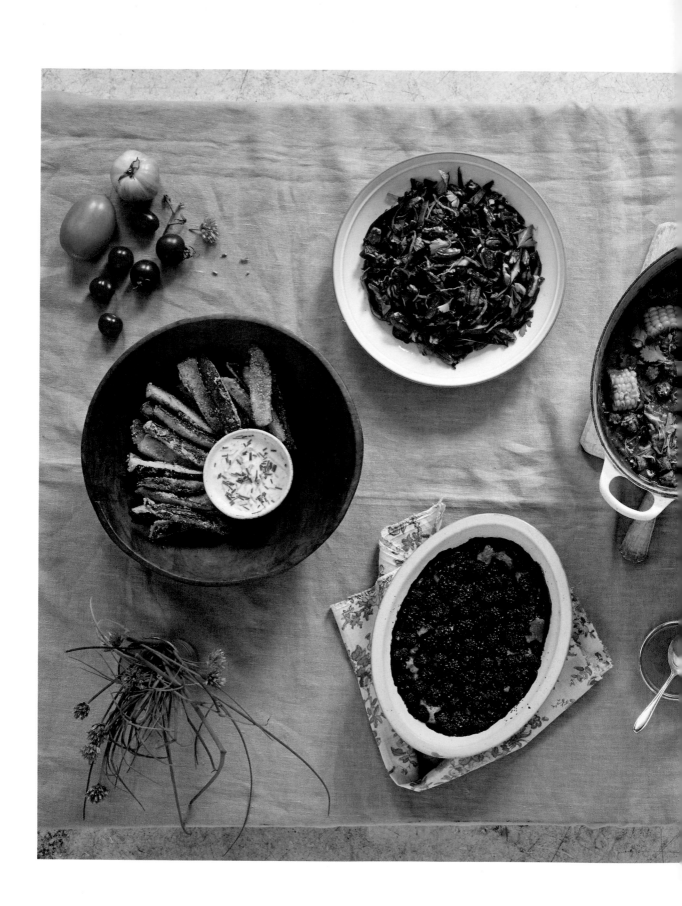

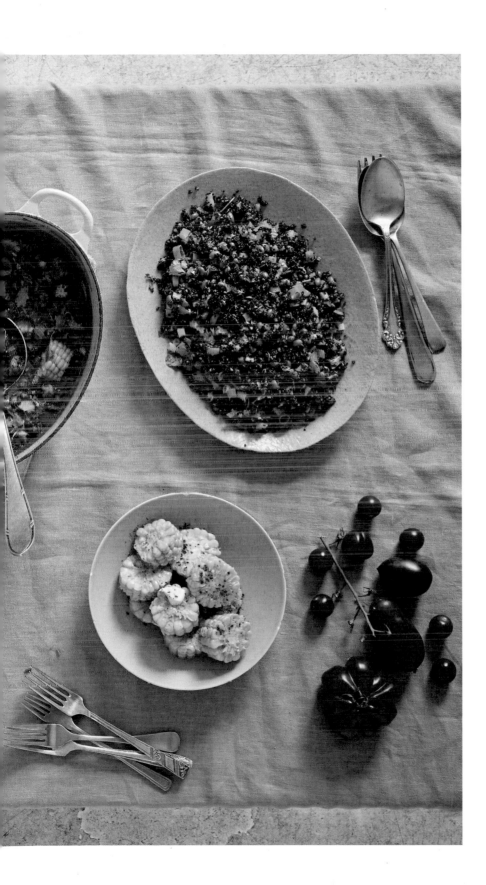

MARDI GRAS SLAW WITH MAPLE PECANS

This slaw is outrageously simple, yet full of flavour, Mardi Gras colours (purple, gold and green) and crunch.

 0.5 PORTION
PER SERVING

PREP   10 MINS
COOK   5 MINS
SERVES   6

1 small red cabbage

⅛ tsp cayenne pepper

zest and juice of 1 lemon

4 tbsp olive oil

2 tbsp maple syrup

a large handful of fresh
   parsley and/or mint,
   finely chopped

a large handful of pecans

sea salt and freshly ground
   black pepper

Finely slice the cabbage, remove the white core and grate the rest. Mix the grated cabbage in a large bowl with a pinch of salt, pepper and just a tiny pinch of cayenne. Add the lemon zest, saving a little to scatter over the top at the end.

Pour 4 tablespoons lemon juice into a clean jam jar with the olive oil and 1 tablespoon of the maple syrup. Shake until thoroughly mixed and looking a little creamy. Mix the dressing into the cabbage and fold in the parsley and/or mint.

Heat a frying pan. Roughly chop the pecans and toast them over a medium heat until fragrant. Add the remaining cayenne and some salt and drizzle with the remaining maple syrup. Mix through until the pecans are sticky and coated.

Crumble the pecans over the top of the cabbage slaw and finish with a grating of lemon zest just before serving.

INSIDE OUT BLACKBERRY COBBLER

There are many styles of cobbler, but this is my favourite. You just make a batter and pile the fruit on top. All the magic happens in the oven, as the batter rises up through the fruit and everything mingles together.

1 PORTION
PER SERVING

PREP   10 MINS
COOK   50 MINS
SERVES   6

75g plain white flour•

½ tsp baking powder

a pinch of sea salt

3 tbsp unsalted butter

100ml maple syrup

1 tsp vanilla extract

½ tsp ground cinnamon

75ml milk

1 tbsp bourbon (optional)

600g blackberries

Preheat the oven to 180°C/Gas 4.

Mix the flour, baking powder and salt in a bowl.

Warm the butter in a saucepan until melted, then add 75ml of the maple syrup, the vanilla, cinnamon and milk and simmer until just warm. Add the bourbon, if using. Whisk the warm milk mixture into the flour and mix gradually until smooth.

Pour the mix into a 23cm baking dish. Scatter the berries over the top of the batter. Drizzle the remaining maple syrup over the berries.

Bake in the centre of the oven for about 40–50 minutes until the batter browns. Leave to cool slightly before serving. Delicious with crème fraîche or vanilla ice cream.

 • *Give it a healthy twist by using wholegrain flour (rye, spelt, kamut or wheat) instead. I prefer it, in fact. It gives it a more rustic texture.*

Persian Feast

In my twenties, I lived near London's Edgware Road. I was surrounded by cafés that lured you in with the sweet, fruity perfume bubbling from ornate shisha pipes, the refreshing smell of fresh mint tea poured from an impossible height, and the whirr of the juicer spinning mountains of exotic fruits into quenching drinks. It was in these little cafés that I experienced my first taste of golden saffron, the soft tickle of rose water in puddings, the elegance of orange blossom. Persian flavours transport you like no other. It could be grey, damp and cold outside, but I was lapping up the warmth of Iran.

As I started to experiment with these flavours in my kitchen at home, I met a wonderful woman called Sepideh Black. Sepi is from Iran and her mother still lives there. Her enthusiasm for the food of her country is simply beautiful. She's a keen gardener, which is evident when you arrive at her London house. There are pots of every variety of mint you can imagine outside, budding pomegranate trees and berries of all shades.

For me, Persian food is all about things from the garden: aromatic herbs, tomatoes, cucumbers, peppers and onions, and all the beautiful fruits: pomegranates, followed by figs, cherries, apricots and melons. While meat certainly has a place in the cuisine, I think the veg dishes on Persian menus always steal the show.

PERSIAN FEAST MENU

Pomegranate Fizz

✳

Fig and Halloumi Skewers with Toasted Sesame and Honey Dressing

✳

Honeyed Aubergine, Feta and Walnut Börek

✳

Roasted Carrot, Lemon and Almond Tagine

Couscous with Griddled Spring Onions

✳

Clementine and Saffron Tea (see page 18)

[THE FULL MENU OFFERS EACH DINER 9.5 PORTIONS]

FIG AND HALLOUMI SKEWERS WITH TOASTED SESAME AND HONEY DRESSING

 2 PORTIONS
PER SERVING

PREP 15 MINS
COOK 30 MINS
SERVES 6

12 smallish fresh figs

a gloss of olive oil

300g halloumi, cut into
  12 cubes

2 tbsp sesame seeds, plus
  an extra pinch for
  sprinkling

1 tbsp runny honey

a handful of fresh mint
  leaves

Preheat the oven to 200°C/Gas 6.

Snip the woody tips of the figs' stems off. Arrange the figs in a roasting tray and roast for 20 minutes on a high shelf, or until the figs are plump, soft and the juices are just starting to come out, creating a sticky syrup.

While the figs are cooking, heat a frying pan and add a gloss of oil. Arrange the halloumi cubes in a single layer and scatter over the sesame seeds. Cook over a low heat until the halloumi has formed a nice golden crust on two sides, and is soft and squidgy in the centre. Remove from the pan and roll the halloumi through the sesame seeds to coat again.

Once the figs are cooked, gloss them with the pan juices, then roll them through any remaining sesame seeds.

Thread the figs and halloumi onto 6 skewers, alternating the figs with the cubes of halloumi sandwiched between them. Drizzle a little shine of honey over the skewers and finish with an extra sprinkling of sesame seeds and mint leaves.

NOTE: If you want to make them in advance and serve warm, reheat in a 200°C/Gas 6 oven for 10 minutes, or until warmed through.

POMEGRANATE FIZZ

 1 JUST UNDER 1 PORTION
PER SERVING

PREP 10 MINS
COOK NIL
SERVES 6

750ml pomegranate juice,
  or 6 fresh pomegranates•

1 tsp rose water

a swirl of honey or a pinch
  of sugar (optional)

750ml champagne or 1 litre
  sparkling water

Mix the juice and rose water. Taste, and whisk in a little honey or sugar if you think it needs it. Chill until ready to serve.

Give the juice a shake, then divide between champagne glasses or long glass tumblers. Top up with champagne or sparkling water. Serve straight away.

• *While there are plenty of places you can buy bottled pomegranate juice, making it fresh is tastier and better for you. You'll need 6 pomegranates to yield about 750ml juice. If you get less, it's no big deal.*

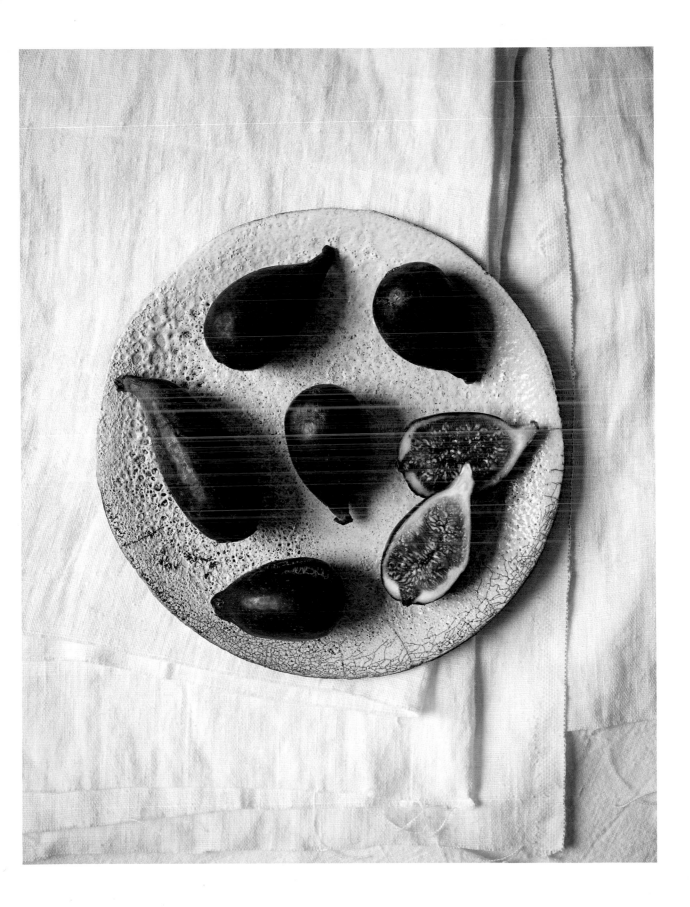

HONEYED AUBERGINE, FETA AND WALNUT BÖREK

1 PORTION PER SERVING

PREP 20 MINS
COOK 1 HOUR
MAKES 9–12

1 aubergine

a few glosses of olive oil

1 onion, thinly sliced

3 tbsp walnuts

a pinch of ground cinnamon

2 tsp honey

6–8 sheets of filo pastry

100g feta, crumbled

a large handful fresh mint leaves, chopped

a dusting of nigella or sesame seeds

sea salt and freshly ground black pepper

Preheat the oven to 200°C/Gas 6.

Halve the aubergine lengthways. Make 1cm-deep cuts into the flesh of the aubergine at 2–3cm intervals on the diagonal. Repeat in the opposite direction to create a criss-cross pattern. Season well. Gloss with olive oil. Bake for 40 minutes, or until tender right the way through and golden on top.

Meanwhile, heat a large frying pan and add a gloss of oil. Add the onions with a pinch of salt and pepper. Cook over a low heat until meltingly tender, about 10 minutes. Mix in the walnuts. Cook a little more, lightly toasting the nuts.

Once the aubergine halves are ready, remove from the oven. Scoop the flesh away from the deep purple skin and roughly chop. Add the aubergine flesh, cinnamon and honey to the onions. Sizzle over a medium heat for a moment – the honey will thicken, giving everything a sweet, sticky gloss. Set aside to cool.

Lay one of the filo pastry sheets on a dry surface. Brush with a thin layer of olive oil. Place another sheet on top. Cut the pastry sheets into three long strips, each about 7cm wide.

Gently mix the crumbled feta and mint into the aubergine filling. Taste. Adjust the seasoning as needed.

Scoop a tablespoon of the filling out. Drop onto the top corner of one of your layered pastry strips. Fold the filled corner over diagonally, making a triangle. Repeat, folding down and then over, while keeping the triangle shape and tucking the filling in each time you fold, until you come to the end of the pastry. Brush with a little oil as you fold.

Repeat with the remaining pastry and filling. You should get 9–12 triangle-shaped pastries.

Place on a lightly oiled baking sheet. Top with a scattering of nigella or sesame seeds. Bake for 15 minutes, or until golden and crisp. Delicious warm or cold. Can be made in advance and reheated.

ROASTED CARROT, LEMON AND ALMOND TAGINE

Roasting carrots to add to your earthy spiced tagine broth is a brilliant manoeuvre, even though this layered approach to cooking totally breaks from tradition. You get extra sweetness from the carrots, with a hint of toastiness.

 4.5 PORTIONS PER SERVING

PREP 20 MINS (PLUS OVERNIGHT SOAKING)

COOK 1 HOUR 20 MINS

SERVES 6

200g split yellow peas

100g dried chickpeas

1 tsp bicarbonate of soda

a few glosses of olive oil

3 garlic cloves, finely chopped

1 tsp ground ginger

1 tsp ground turmeric

1 tsp ground cumin

1 tsp ground cinnamon

a pinch of chilli flakes (more or less, to taste), plus extra chilli flakes, to serve

250g tomatoes, diced

50g dried apricots, finely chopped

1 litre veg or chicken stock

500g shallots

500g carrots

zest and juice of 1 lemon

a large handful almonds, roughly chopped and toasted

2 large handfuls of fresh coriander and/or mint

sea salt and ground pepper

Tumble the split peas and chickpeas into a large, lidded pan. Cover with water. Swirl in the bicarbonate of soda. Pop a lid on. Soak overnight.

The next day, drain the soaking peas. Rinse. Set aside.

Rinse your large pan. Place over a medium heat. Add a gloss of oil to the warmed pan. Lower the heat. Swirl in the garlic and tomatoes. Sizzle until they cook down to a paste.

Swirl in the spices and chopped apricots. Cook for a second, just until fragrant. Fold in your rinsed peas. Pour in the stock. Bring to the boil.

Skim off any frothy bits. Give it a stir. Pop a lid on. Turn the heat right down. Simmer for 1 hour.

Meanwhile, preheat the oven to 220°C/Gas 7. Place a large roasting tin in the oven to heat up. Bring the kettle or a pan of water on to boil. Place the shallots in a pan and cover with the boiling water. Soak them while you halve or quarter the carrots lengthways, or leave whole if they're small. Drain the shallots. Strip off the peel. Leave them whole if small, or halve/quarter if they're larger.

Tumble the carrots and shallots into the warmed roasting tin. Dust with a little salt and pepper, gloss with oil and give everything a mix to nicely coat. Roast for 45 minutes, or until the carrots and onions are tender and nicely coloured.

Add lemon zest and juice to the split peas. Taste. Season and add more spice, as needed. Once the carrots and shallots are cooked, fold a pinch of chilli through the mix. Pile them on top of your split pea tagine. Keep warm until ready to serve, or if making in advance, chill and reheat before serving.

Scatter the coriander and toasted almonds over the top just before serving. I like to have a little pot of chilli flakes alongside the tagine in case people want to crank up the heat.

COUSCOUS WITH GRIDDLED SPRING ONIONS

 1 PORTION
PER SERVING

PREP   5 MINS
COOK   20 MINS
SERVES 6

1 mug of couscous

2 mugs of boiling water

500g spring onions

2 handfuls of fresh mint

200g feta

a drizzle of olive oil

sea salt and freshly ground
   black pepper

Put the couscous in a lidded pan or a bowl you can cover. Add a pinch of salt and the water. Stir through, pop a lid on and leave for 10 minutes, or until all the water is absorbed.

Cut the spring onions on the diagonal into roughly 3cm hunks.

Heat a large frying pan or griddle until smoking hot. No oil is needed. Rinse the spring onions, then toss them into the hot pan with a little water still clinging to them. Arrange in a single layer, add a pinch of salt and pepper, and fry them, turning often, until slightly charred around the edges. Tumble onto a plate.

Fluff up the couscous with a fork. Fold in the spring onions and a handful of the fresh mint. Crumble the feta over the top and gently mix through. Finish with the remaining mint and a drizzle of olive oil. Taste, and add a little more salt and pepper, if needed.

Delicious alongside the Roasted Carrot, Lemon and Almond Tagine (see page 175).

Medieval Feast

The best way to lure me into a history lesson is through food. When I moved to England nearly two decades ago, one of the first places I visited was Hampton Court Palace, former stomping ground of King Henry VIII. I was immediately seduced by the Palace kitchens. Large wooden bowls are set along the enormous heavy tables, brimming with fresh thyme, rosemary, sage and parsley. There's the fierce heat of a roaring fire, where whole animals, speared on metal rods, would have been roasted above the flames. There were mustardy cabbages and aniseedy fennel, plucked from the Palace's kitchen garden (now resurrected and open to the public). The kitchen was where you got a real taste of history.

I returned to the Palace recently with my son to see the forgotten chocolate kitchens. They'd just opened after nearly 300 years languishing as a store room. It was during King George I's rein that chocolate swept the country off its feet and the King recruited his own personal chocolatier. Thomas Tosier, the Willy Wonka of his day, who took up residence in the Palace.

Winding our way through the Palace to find Tosier's quarters, we encountered a tome which gave us a further bite of history: *The Medieval Cookbook* by Maggie Black.

I devoured Maggie's book on our way home. The sheer number of beautiful and inspiring vegetable dishes in it took me by surprise, as wealthy nobles viewed fresh fruit and veg with suspicion. In its pure form, they thought it to be riddled with pests and disease. Food that came from the ground was only seen fit to feed the poor.

The following menu celebrates the vegetable dishes of the era, marrying the exotic and expensive spice potions Henry VIII would have feasted on.

MEDIEVAL FEAST MENU

~

Mushroom Pasties

*

Pork Roast with Spiced Wine and Shallots

Medieval Braised Greens

Winter Pickles

*

Honeyed Fig Pastries

[THE FULL MENU OFFERS EACH DINER 5.5
PORTIONS]

MUSHROOM PASTIES

These pasties are like giant pastry ravioli. They're a perfect table setting for a decadent feast.

1 PORTION
PER SERVING

PREP 20 MINS, PLUS CHILLING
COOK 35 MINS
MAKES 8 PASTIES

400g wholegrain (spelt, wheat or kamut) or buckwheat flour, plus extra for dusting

½ tsp sea salt

½ tsp finely ground dried rosemary (optional)

200g cold butter, cubed

1 egg, separated

8–12 tbsp cold water

500g button or chestnut mushrooms

2 tsp Dijon mustard

a good pinch of freshly ground black pepper

100g Cheddar or similar cheese, grated

Preheat the oven to 200°C/Gas 6. Lightly oil a large baking tray.

Mix the flour, salt, rosemary, if using, and baking powder together. Cut the butter into 1-2cm cubes. Bit by bit add them to the flour. Coat the butter in flour as you add them. Rub the butter into the flour until it resembles breadcrumbs. Add the egg yolk and enough water (adding it 1 tbsp at a time) to bring it together into a soft, silky (not sticky) dough.

On a floured surface, pat the dough into a rectangle. Roll until 1–2cm thick. Fold in the sides like you're folding a letter. Rotate the rectangle 90 degrees. Roll out again. Repeat this five times, ending with a letter-folded piece of dough. Wrap up in a clean tea towel. Refrigerate for 30 minutes.

Bring a pan of salted water to the boil and plunge the mushrooms into the water for a minute. Drain and pat the mushrooms dry, then thinly slice them and place them in a bowl with the mustard, pepper and cheese.

Divide the dough into 16 pieces. Roll the pieces into balls. On a generously floured surface roll one of the balls of pastry into a circle.

Whisk the egg white. Brush the outer rim of the pastry with the beaten egg. Spoon a mound of the mushroom mix in the centre, leaving 2–3cm rim of pastry around the edge. Roll out another circle of pastry. Place it on top. Use your index finger to seal the pastry around the rim you painted with egg. Use a large circle cutter or the rim of a large glass or bowl as a guide to help you trim off the rough edges of the round pastry.

Crimp the edges with a fork or your fingers. Use a spatula to transfer the pasty to the baking tray. Repeat with the remaining pastry until you have 8 pasties. Brush the tops with remaining egg white and cut a cross in the pastry top to let steam out.

Bake the pasties for 25–30 minutes or until golden on top.

● *I think the added texture and nuttiness of a wholegrain flour works beautifully with the mushroom filling. If you're gluten-free, buckwheat flour is a great option.*

PORK ROAST WITH SPICED WINE AND SHALLOTS

In medieval times, the pork would have been skewered on a long metal rod and cooked over an enormous spit, with some poor soul in charge of turning and basting the meat until beautifully cooked. I don't think I'm taking a wild leap of faith by guessing that most people don't have a spit in their kitchen. But with all the spices and a beautiful piece of meat, you can certainly evoke a taste of the day.

 PORTION PER SERVING

PREP   15 MINS, PLUS RESTING
COOK   2½ HOURS
SERVES 6

500g shallots or onions

1.5kg pork shoulder joint

1½ tsp ground coriander

1 tsp caraway seeds

½ tsp freshly ground black pepper

1 garlic clove, finely minced

2 tsp runny honey

250ml red wine

a good pinch of sea salt

250ml chicken or veg stock

Preheat the oven to 220°C/Gas 7.

Peel the shallots and halve or quarter them if they're on the large side. If using onions, peel and cut into 2–3cm-thick wedges.

Cut a criss-cross pattern into the pork fat, just cutting fat, not the meat.

Lay the pork on a double sheet of foil large enough to enclose it, fat-side up, in a roasting tray. Arrange the shallots/onions around it.

In a bowl, whisk the coriander, caraway and black pepper with the garlic, honey and wine. Pour this around the sides of the joint and seal the foil securely. If you're out of foil, just put the meat and spiced wine in a lidded casserole dish (although the meat is more tender when cooked in foil). Place the pork in the oven. Immediately lower the heat to 160°C/Gas 3. Cook for 30 minutes for every 500g, so for a 1.5kg joint, cook for 1½ hours. Adjust the cooking time according to the size of your joint.

At the end of the cooking time, crank the heat back up to 220°C/Gas 7. Uncover the pork a little to reveal the fat. Sprinkle a generous pinch or two of salt over the fat and cook for another 25 minutes at this high heat, or until the fat is nicely crisped and golden.

Remove from the oven. Pierce the pork with the point of a knife and press the meat. If the juices run clear, the meat is done. If the juices are red, lower the heat to 160°C/Gas 3 and cook for a further 30 minutes, or until the juices run clear.

Rest the meat for at least 30 minutes to 1 hour before carving. If the crackling isn't quite crisp enough, carefully cut the fat off, trying not to cut into the meat, and slice into strips. Lay on a roasting tray and pop into a 200°C/Gas 6 oven, checking often, until golden and crisp.

To make a gravy, tip the cooking juices into a frying pan over a medium-high heat and reduce them down with the stock until the flavour is concentrated and rich. Add more wine or honey, if needed.

Keep the onions in the foil parcel to stay warm. Arrange them around the pork or in a dish to serve up alongside the meat. Strain the gravy through a sieve and serve warm with the pork and shallots or onions.

MEDIEVAL BRAISED GREENS

I served these greens to friends for Sunday lunch and they disappeared before the meat, which demonstrates the magical powers of a little pinch of sugar and spice.

 1 PORTION
PER SERVING

PREP 5 MINS
COOK 10 MINS
SERVES 6

500g spring greens, kale
  or Savoy cabbage

a splash of olive oil

a pinch of grated nutmeg
  and ground cinnamon

1 tsp brown sugar or honey

sea salt and ground pepper

Wash the greens and trim off any woody stems or cores.

Heat a large pan on the hob over a high heat. Add a splash of water to the pan, enough to create a 2.5cm-deep puddle. Plunge the greens into the pot with a good pinch of salt and pepper, and quickly fold them through the water in the pot, getting them evenly moistened. Cook for 5 minutes or until just softened to a bright, glossy grain. Drain.

Return the pan to the heat (wipe it dry if it's still damp). Add a splash of oil, then tumble in the greens, along with a good pinch of nutmeg and cinnamon and the sugar or honey. Fold through and taste, adding a little salt, pepper and more sugar and spice, as needed. Serve warm alongside a pie or a Sunday roast.

WINTER PICKLES

2.5 PORTIONS
PER JAR

PREP 20 MINS, PLUS SOAKING
COOK 20 MINS
MAKES 4 x 330 ML JARS

650g mix of turnips, carrots,
  celery and/or white cabbage

250g firm pears

3 tbsp sea salt

½ tsp ground ginger

a pinch of saffron

200ml cider vinegar

2 tbsp currants or raisins

300ml cider

5 tbsp runny honey

½ tsp Dijon mustard

⅛ tsp ground cinnamon

⅛ tsp freshly ground pepper

1 star anise

⅛ tsp fennel seeds

Bring a big pot of water to the boil. Thinly slice the veg, and core and shred the white cabbage. Plunge the veg into the water.

Peel, core and slice the pears into 2cm hunks. Add to the veg. Cook until the veg and fruit just soften. Drain.

Spread the veg and fruit into the base of a shallow glass dish (avoid metal as the salt will make it rust).

Sprinkle with the salt, ginger, saffron and 2 tablespoons of the vinegar. Mix through. Cover and leave overnight (or for 12 hours).

Drain and rinse well, then add the currants. Pack into sterilised storage jars, with at least 2.5cm free space at the top of the jars.

Pour the cider into a pan. Swirl in the honey. Bring to a simmer. Skim any froth bubbling at the surface.

Add the remaining vinegar, the mustard and spices.

Reduce the heat and stir without boiling until the honey has fully dissolved into the liquid.

Bring to the boil. When it's piping hot, pour over the vegetables, covering with 1cm of the liquid. Secure with vinegar-proof seals. Chill before serving. Store extra jars at room temperature for up to 6 months. Eat within 2 weeks once opened.

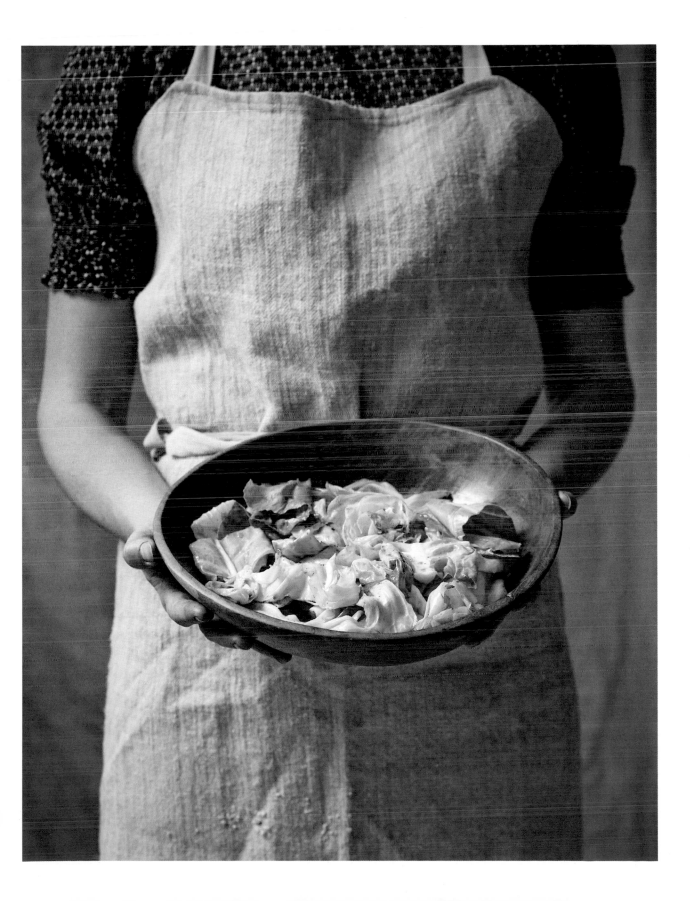

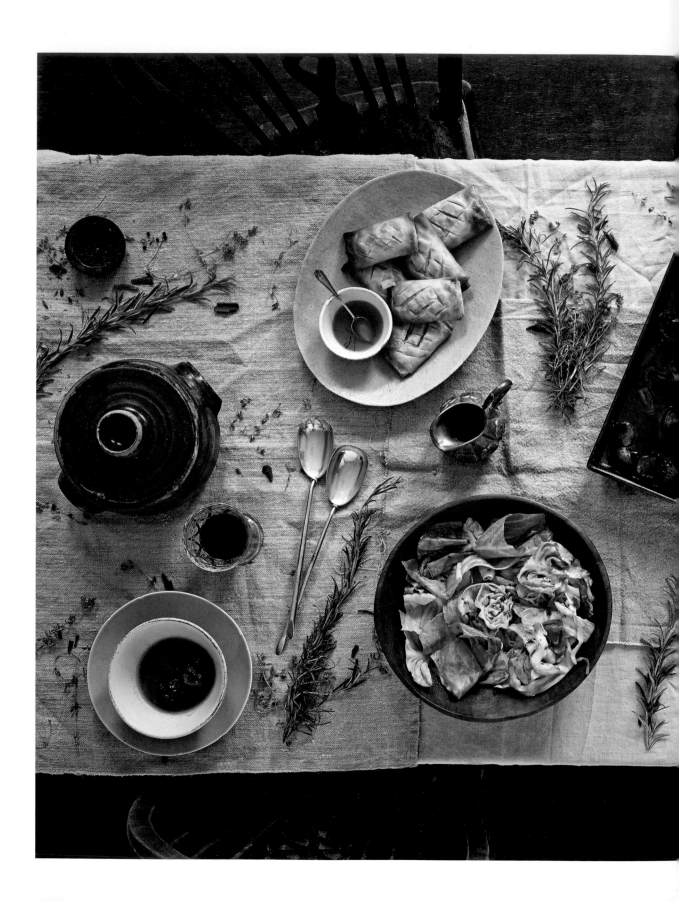

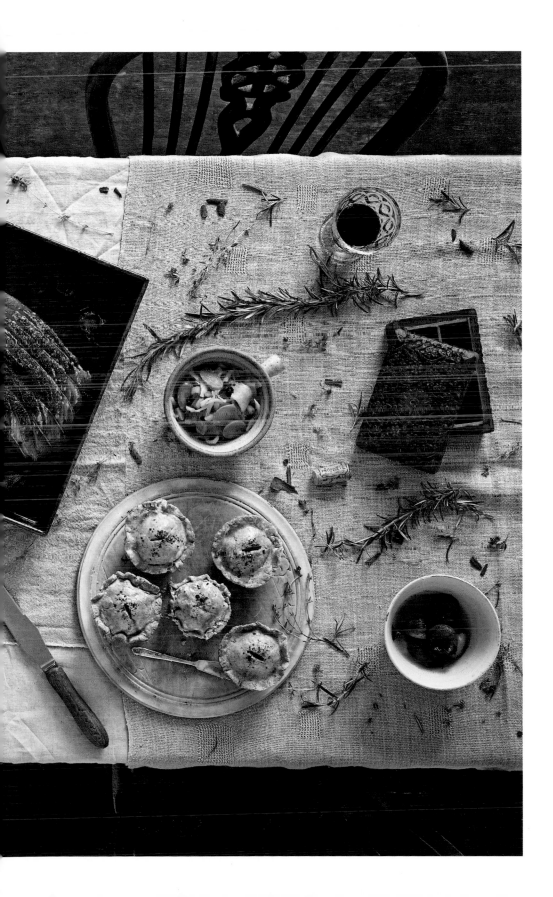

HONEYED FIG PASTRIES

The original fig rolls. Delicious warm, I like to prepare them in advance and then pop them in to cook while I'm clearing the main course and making the coffee. Beautiful with a cardamom-infused coffee or a rose-petal tea to wash them down.

 PORTION PER SERVING

PREP 20 MINS
COOK 15 MINS
MAKES 6

12 dried figs, roughly chopped

100ml water

a good pinch of saffron strands

⅛ tsp ground ginger

⅛ tsp ground cloves

6 sheets of filo pastry

2–3 tbsp butter, melted (for vegans, use olive or coconut oil)

water or beaten egg, for brushing

3 tbsp honey or maple syrup

sea salt and freshly ground black pepper

Preheat the oven to 200°C/Gas 6.

Place the figs in a saucepan with the water. Bring to the boil, then lower the heat and simmer until they're tender and plump.

Pour the water off the figs into a small saucepan. Spoon 2 tablespoons of the warm fig liquid into a dish and mix with the saffron.

In a blender or food processor, purée the warm figs with the ginger, cloves, soaked saffron strands (including soaking water) and a pinch of salt and pepper.

Lay a sheet of filo pastry on a cutting board. Lightly brush with melted butter then lay a second layer on top. Brush lightly with butter then set a third sheet on top and brush with more butter. Cut your layered pastry into 3 long, equally sized strips (each about 7cm wide).

Dollop a large rounded tablespoon of the fig purée at the top of each strip. Roll the pastry, starting with the filled end, making a little envelope-style parcel full of fig. Press the open sides of the parcel to seal it as you roll. Cut a couple of diagonal slits on the top of each. If necessary, brush with a little water or beaten egg to seal, if needed. Repeat with the remaining pastry and filling.

Brush the base and sides of a baking dish with a little butter. Arrange the filled pastries in the dish and bake for 15 minutes, or until puffed up and golden.

While they cook, boil the remaining fig soaking liquid until reduced. Swirl in the honey or maple syrup and cook for a little longer, just enough to warm through and thicken a touch more.

Serve the pastries with the warmed fig syrup.

Caribbean Feast

Oh, how I'd love to be basking in the Barbados sun, walking barefoot on the beach with the hot sand beneath my feet. The Caribbean is a place I've longed to visit, and its cuisine is something I've only experienced through friends cooking up their memories.

My friend Alison McNaught dreamt up the following menu, fresh from a Caribbean yoga break. Ali runs and cooks up a storm in one of my favourite local cafés, Domali.

The menu was created to celebrate a fruit many of us probably take for granted: the banana. It sits in just about everyone's fruit bowl, we slice it up for our cereal, eat it on the run, tuck into sandwiches with a slick of sticky peanut butter, or split it in half for one of my all-time favourite ice cream dishes: the mighty banana split.

The future of bananas, and many tropical ingredients we now take for granted like coffee, chocolate and nuts, are threatened by price wars. Banana producer Alexis Martinez Palacios joined us in Domali for our Caribbean-themed feast to tell us how supporting Fairtrade, or even sourcing direct from suppliers, makes a huge difference to the livelihood of the farmers.

Our dinner was held at the end of February, during a period British farmers call the Hungry Gap. It's when the last of their winter stores are running out and the first of their new crops have yet to feed through. Even though it's the leanest time of year, we managed to create a menu full of rich, exciting local flavours brought further to life by marrying them with a kiss of sunshine from Fairtrade farms abroad. The following recipes are a taste of our memorable meal with Alexis.

CARIBBEAN FEAST MENU

~

Winter Roots and Leaves with Tropical Dressing

*

Ali's Caribbean Curry with Coconut-crusted Fish

Lime and Thyme Rice

Raw Banana Chutney

*

Rebel's Hop Banoffee

[THE FULL MENU OFFERS EACH DINER 8.5 PORTIONS]

WINTER ROOTS AND LEAVES WITH TROPICAL DRESSING

2 PORTIONS
PER SERVING

PREP   20 MINS
COOK   NIL
SERVES 6

200g fresh pineapple,
   coarsely grated

4 tbsp olive or rapeseed oil
   (or a 50: 50 mix)

1 tbsp freshly grated ginger

¼ tsp ground allspice

a pinch of chilli powder

500g colourful root veg●

250g winter salad leaves,
   washed

100g Brazil nuts, thinly
   sliced

sea salt and freshly ground
   black pepper

Place the grated pineapple in a bowl and swirl in the oil, ginger, allspice, a pinch of chilli powder and a pinch of salt and pepper. Mix well to create a sort of chunky dressing. Taste, and tweak the seasoning, as needed.

Peel or scrub the root veg clean, then use a veg peeler or mandolin to carve the veg into wispy ribbons. Pile these on top of the pineapple dressing and mix through; get your hands in there – it's much more fun.

Just before serving, arrange the winter leaves over the top, gently mix through, and finish with the toasted nuts.

● *Try to go for a rainbow of colours: beetroot, carrots and celeriac are lovely; even better if you can get a mix of beetroot (golden, Chioggia) and carrot (purple, yellow, red) varieties.*

ALI'S CARIBBEAN CURRY

What keeps me coming back to Domali is the café's beautiful homemade food. Everything is earthy, comforting, and there's a real focus on seasonal vegetables, just as with this gorgeous curry, for which Ali kindly shared the recipe.

 PORTIONS PER SERVING

PREP 20 MINS
COOK 40 MINS
SERVES 6

5 garlic cloves, finely minced

75g fresh ginger, finely grated

1 Scotch Bonnet or red hot chilli (more or less, to taste)

a few glosses of oil

2 onions, finely chopped

2 sticks of celery, thinly sliced

1 green pepper, thinly sliced (seeds and stem removed)

1 star anise ground to a powder or 2 whole

1 cinnamon stick

2 bay leaves

1 tbsp tomato purée

400ml coconut milk

500ml veg stock

750g dense butternut (or similar) squash or sweet potato, chopped into 2–3cm chunks

1 tbsp fresh thyme leaves

75g curly kale, thinly shredded

a pinch of ground allspice

¼ tsp freshly grated nutmeg

Finely chop or blitz the garlic, ginger and chillies until they form a paste.

Heat a large pan and add a gloss of oil. Add the chilli paste, followed by the chopped onions and celery. Cook until translucent.

Fold in the sliced green peppers. Add the star anise, cinnamon stick and bay leaves. Sizzle for a moment. Swirl in the tomato purée.

Pour in the coconut milk and stock. Increase the heat to medium. When the liquid is bubbling, add the squash or sweet potato and the thyme leaves. Cook the curry for 30 minutes, or until the squash is just tender.

When the squash is ready, plunge the sliced kale into the pot along with the allspice. Cook until just tender. Taste. Tweak the seasoning as needed. Finish with a dusting of nutmeg before serving.

COCONUT CRUSTED FISH

Place 6 large or 12 smaller white skinless fish fillets on a large plate. Sprinkle with salt and pepper and the zest of a lime. Squeeze the juice of the lime over, giving it a good soaking. On another plate, mix ½ a mug of plain white or gluten-free white flour and ½ a mug of desiccated coconut. Press the fish fillets into the mix, one by one, coating them on both sides.

Heat a large frying pan until smoking hot. Add enough oil to create a thin film, then add the fish and sizzle until golden, about 2 minutes on each side. Do this in batches, if needed, as you don't want to crowd the pan. Finish with a touch of sea salt. This will serve 6. Serve on a large platter with lime wedges and alongside Ali's Caribbean Curry.

LIME AND THYME RICE

PORTION PER SERVING

PREP   5 MINS
COOK   25 MINS
SERVES 6

1 mug of brown rice

2 garlic cloves, chopped

a gloss of oil

2 mugs of water or stock

2 x 400g tins of kidney beans

zest and juice of 2 limes

1 tbsp fresh thyme leaves

sea salt and freshly ground black pepper

Heat a large lidded pan and add the rice. Swirl in the garlic and add a gloss of oil and a pinch of salt and pepper. Pour in the water or stock, pop a lid on, and cook for 20 minutes, or until all the liquid is fully absorbed. Remove from the heat, lid still on, and leave to steam for a further 10 minutes.

In a separate pan, warm the beans in their cooking juices. Drain the beans then mix them through the rice. Add the lime zest and juice along with the fresh thyme leaves, taste, and adjust the seasoning, as needed.

RAW BANANA CHUTNEY

A sweet and gently spiced chutney that's wonderfully refreshing with Ali's Caribbean Curry and the Coconut Crusted Fish, pages (see pages 186–187).

PORTION PER SERVING

PREP   15 MINS
COOK   NIL
SERVES 6

3 dates, pitted

1 tbsp freshly grated pineapple

1 lime, zest and 1 tsp juice

¼ tsp ground allspice

¼ tsp ground ginger

3 cardamom pods, seeds finely ground

½ red chilli, finely chopped

2 large bananas

sea salt and freshly ground black pepper

Finely chop your dates. Tumble them into a bowl with the pineapple, lime zest and juice, spices and fresh chilli.

Peel the bananas. Finely dice. Fold into the other ingredients. Season with salt and pepper, to taste. Add more spices or lime, as you wish.

Best served straight away.

REBEL'S HOP BANOFFEE

I may be in dangerous waters here, but I've attempted to give the classic banoffee pie a healthy makeover. I bumped into a friend before heading to my kitchen to attempt the feat. She laughed at the idea, but everyone who tried it gave it a resounding thumbs up.

 1.5 PORTIONS
PER SERVING

PREP	20 MINS (PLUS OVERNIGHT STRAINING)
COOK	10 MINS
SERVES	6

½ tsp vanilla extract, or seeds from ½ a vanilla pod

1 tbsp icing sugar

a pinch of sea salt

2 x 500g tubs of coconut yoghurt•

3–4 bananas, cut into 1–2cm thick hunks

a grating of fresh nutmeg (optional)

a dusting of cocoa powder, to finish

FOR THE BASE
200g cashew nuts, toasted

1 tsp ground cinnamon

½ tsp sea salt

150g pitted dates

FOR THE TOFFEE
200g pitted dates

2 tbsp water

2 tbsp rum (optional; use strongly brewed coffee in place of rum for a booze-free pie)

200ml coconut milk

For the cream: swirl the vanilla, sugar and a good pinch of sea salt into the coconut milk or yoghurt. Taste. Add more sugar, if needed. Line a sieve with a clean muslin cloth or tea towel and set it over a bowl. Pour the milk or yoghurt in the centre of the cloth. Bring the sides of the cloth together, pulling it up like a drawstring handbag to cradle it. Tie it with string. Rest it in the sieve, placed over a bowl, and let it refrigerate overnight – the whey from the yoghurt will drain, giving you a thick coconut yoghurt cream.

For the base: grind the cashew nuts with the cinnamon, salt and dates in a blender or food processor until it all comes together to form a sticky ball. Press this into the base of a round 23cm springform pan with a removable base. The base should be about 1cm thick. If it's more than this, remove some of the mix to make it thinner; you can freeze or snack on the excess.

For the toffee: warm the dates in a pan with the water and rum or coffee until they soften, about 5 minutes. Whizz to a fine paste in a food processor or blender, then whisk in the coconut milk. Return to the pan and gently heat, stirring often, until thickened and toffee-like, about 5 minutes. Cool a little before slathering over the cashew base.

Dot the banana slices on top of the toffee, in a single or double layer depending on how thick you've sliced them. Dust with a little fresh grated nutmeg, if using.

Spread the thickened coconut yoghurt over the top of the tart.

Chill for at least 1 hour before serving, then finish with a dusting of cocoa powder.

> • *For the topping, you can either use coconut-flavoured cow's milk yoghurt, or for a dairy free option, seek yoghurt made with coconut milk, like CoYo.*

TREATS

Ice Crème

THE BASICS: The following recipes are totally effort-free. You don't even need an ice-cream maker. If you put the mix in a shallow metal container (the metal gets it colder faster), you can have delicious homemade, no-churn, sugar-free ice cream in about an hour. The ice cream on its own, of course, doesn't help you notch up fruit and veg servings, but pair it with some fresh fruit and you're getting somewhere. The secret ingredient here is crème fraîche, but do opt for the full-fat version. It freezes beautifully, stays creamy and, once frozen, will keep for up to a month.

CINNAMON TAHINI WITH NECTARINES

PORTION PER SERVING

PREP	15 MINS (PLUS 1–2 HOURS' FREEZING)
COOK	2–5 MINS
SERVES	4

4 tbsp runny honey

⅛ tsp ground cinnamon

4 egg yolks

300g full fat crème fraîche

1 tbsp tahini

4 ripe nectarines, sliced

Place the honey and cinnamon in a small pan over a low heat and gently warm through. Remove from the heat.

Put the egg yolks in a large bowl and pour in the warm honey. Whisk until the eggs and honey are thick and creamy, around 5 minutes. Leave the mixture to cool, then slowly work in the crème fraîche and tahini until smooth and creamy.

Pour into individual ramekins or a shallow metal dish. Freeze for 1–2 hours or until set. Remove from the freezer a few minutes before serving with fresh nectarine slices.

SALTED DOUBLE CHOCOLATE ALMOND WITH RASPBERRIES

 PORTION PER SERVING

PREP   15 MINS (PLUS 1–2 HOURS' FREEZING)

COOK   2–5 MINS

SERVES 4

4 tbsp runny honey

4 egg yolks

300g full-fat crème fraîche

2 tsp cocoa powder

35g dark chocolate, melted

a good pinch of sea salt

2 tbsp flaked almonds, toasted

350g raspberries

Place the honey in a small pan over a low heat and gently warm through. Remove from the heat.

Put the egg yolks in a large bowl and pour in the warm honey. Whisk until the eggs and honey are thick and creamy, around 5 minutes. Leave the mixture to cool, then slowly work in the crème fraîche and cocoa powder until smooth and creamy. Fold the melted chocolate, a good pinch of sea salt and toasted almonds through the mix. Taste. Add a little more salt, if you like.

Pour into individual ramekins or a shallow metal dish. Freeze for 1–2 hours or until set. Remove from the freezer a few minutes before serving with fresh raspberries.

SAFFRON WITH STRAWBERRIES OR RHUBARB

 PORTION PER SERVING

PREP   15 MINS (PLUS 1–2 HOURS' FREEZING)

COOK   2–5 MINS

SERVES 4

4 tbsp runny honey

a good pinch of saffron strands

4 egg yolks

300g full-fat crème fraîche

350g ripe strawberries or rhubarb

Place the honey and saffron in a small pan over a low heat and gently warm through. Remove from the heat.

Put the egg yolks in a large bowl and pour in the warm honey. Whisk until the eggs and honey are thick and creamy, around 5 minutes. Leave the mixture to cool, then slowly work in the crème fraîche until smooth and creamy.

Pour into individual ramekins or a shallow metal dish. Freeze for 1–2 hours or until set. Remove from the freezer a few minutes before serving with fresh strawberries or cooked rhubarb.

> **COOKED RHUBARB**
> Cut the rhubarb into 2cm chunks. Place in a saucepan with enough water to come halfway up the rhubarb. Simmer gently until tender, adding more water if needed. Swirl in a little honey, sugar or your favourite sweetener, to taste. Serve the rhubarb warm or cold.

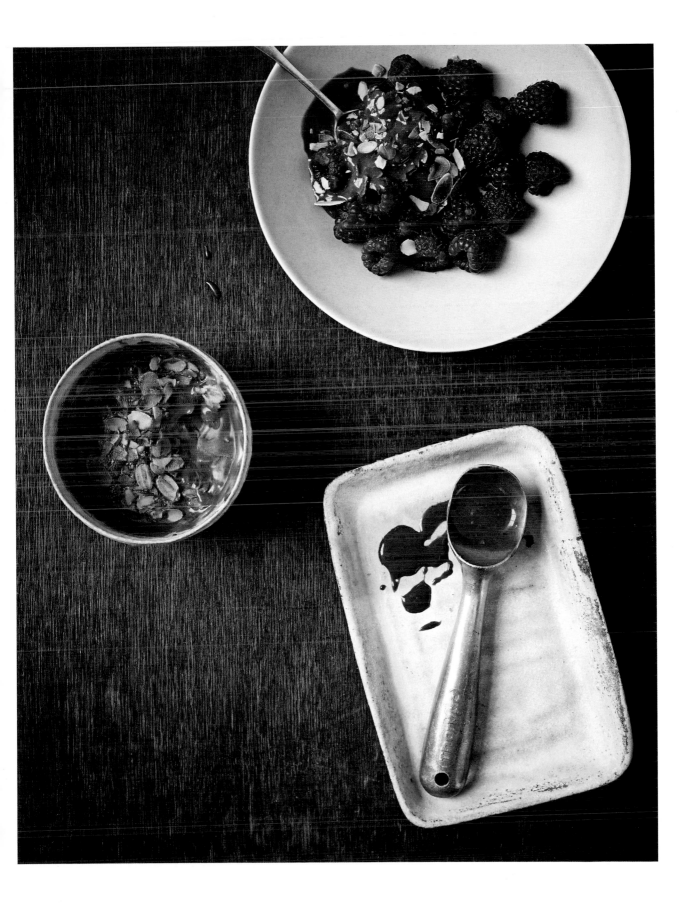

GINGERBREAD WITH PEACH OR ROASTED APPLE

 PORTION PER SERVING

PREP	15 MINS (PLUS 1–2 HOURS' FREEZING)
COOK	2–5 MINS
SERVES	4

3 tbsp treacle

½ tsp ground cinnamon

½ tsp ginger

¼ tsp ground cloves

4 egg yolks

300g full-fat crème fraîche

4 ripe peaches, halved and stoned, or 4 roasted apples•

Place the treacle and spices in a small pan over a low heat and gently warm through. Remove from the heat.

Put the egg yolks in a large bowl and pour in the warm spiced treacle. Whisk until the eggs and treacle are thick and creamy, around 5 minutes. Leave the mixture to cool, then slowly work in the crème fraîche until smooth and creamy.

Pour into individual ramekins or a shallow metal dish. Freeze for 1–2 hours or until set. Remove from the freezer a few minutes before serving with halved peaches or roasted apples.

• *See the Roasted Apple with Honey Nutmeg Toasts recipe on page 52 for tips on how to roast your apples.*

FENNEL SEED AND CHILLI WITH LATE SUMMER FRUIT

 PORTION PER SERVING

PREP	15 MINS (PLUS 1–2 HOURS FREEZING)
COOK	2–5 MINS
SERVES	4

4 tbsp runny honey

1 tsp fennel seeds, toasted

a pinch of chilli flakes (more or less, to taste)

seeds from ½ a vanilla pod or 1 tsp vanilla extract

4 egg yolks

300g full-fat crème fraîche

350g ripe plums, blackberries or figs

Place the honey, fennel seeds, chilli and vanilla in a small pan over a low heat and gently warm through. Remove from the heat.

Put the egg yolks in a large bowl and pour in the warm honey. Whisk until the eggs and honey are thick and creamy, around 5 minutes. Leave the mixture to cool, then slowly work in the crème fraîche until smooth and creamy.

Pour into individual ramekins or a shallow metal dish. Freeze for 1–2 hours or until set. Remove from the freezer a few minutes before serving with fresh plums, blackberries or figs.

Cake

THE BASICS: Over the years, I've spent a lot of time in my kitchen, playing with cake recipes to see if I could give them nips and tucks here and there to lighten the sugar and butter. Sometimes these experiments don't quite work, but they're always edible, even if they've sunk in the middle or have turned out a little squidgy. Below are some tips to ensure you have cake success, but if it all goes wrong don't fret. Mistakes are what makes an experienced cook, and a bit of cream or icing and fruit on top is the perfect plaster to cover up any cake wounds.

ONE: Always bake your cake on the middle shelf in the centre of the oven. This is where the heat is most even.

TWO: Don't try to cook 10 cakes at once. I've tried this and it doesn't work. You can, however, bake 2 tins of cake side by side on the same shelf in as central a position as possible.

THREE: Fill the cake tin no more than three-quarters full. Any more than this and it's likely to overflow.

FOUR: Some cooks say the size of eggs matters, but I get mine from a farm and they don't sort their eggs into sizes; I just use what I've got. Most eggs are around 50g in weight, so if you're unsure, crack your egg into a dish and weigh up 50g for each egg called for in a recipe.

FIVE: Don't leave your cake in the oven to cool. It tends to sink in the middle when you do.

SIX: Let your cake cool fully before removing it from the tin. It should shrink from the sides a little. If you remove or cut into it when it's hot, it's likely to fall apart or be a little gooey inside. Allowing the residual heat and steam to work their way through is part of the final cooking process. This is a vital tip for success with the muffin recipes in the Breakfast section (see pages 11–16).

CINNAMON PARSNIP LAYERED SPONGE WITH BROWN BUTTER ICING

This deliciously moist sponge proves that veg most certainly has a place in cakes.

0.5 PORTION
PER SERVING

PREP 20 MINS
COOK 30 MINS
SERVES 10

250g parsnips, peeled and coarsely grated

1 apple, coarsely grated

zest and juice of 1 lemon

250g plain white flour

250g caster sugar

1 tbsp ground cinnamon, plus extra for topping

1 tsp ground ginger

1 tbsp baking powder

½ tsp bicarbonate of soda

100g runny honey

100ml warm water or apple juice

150ml olive oil

3 eggs

250g butter

300g icing sugar

a large handful almonds, to decorate (optional)

sea salt

Preheat the oven to 180°C/Gas 4. Oil two 23cm round cake tins with removable bases and line the bottom of each one with baking parchment.

In a bowl, mix the grated parsnips and apple with the lemon zest and juice. Set aside.

In a second bowl, mix the flour, sugar, spices, baking powder and bicarbonate of soda. Fold the parsnip and apple mix through the spiced flour.

Whisk the honey and water together until the honey dissolves. Add the oil, crack in the eggs and whisk everything together. Pour the eggy mix over the flour mix and gently fold through, being careful not to overmix.

Divide the batter between the tins. Bake on the middle shelf of the oven for 30 minutes, or until the cakes are golden on top and fully set in the centre. Insert a skewer to test – if it comes out clean, they're done. Remove from the oven and leave to cool before removing from the tins.

For the icing, melt the butter in a large saucepan until frothy. When it turns from golden yellow to a light, nutty-smelling brown, remove from the heat. Sift in the icing sugar and whisk (ideally with a hand mixer) until smooth and creamy.

Transfer one of the cooled cakes to a plate or cake stand. Smooth half the icing over and top with the second cake. Smooth the remaining icing over the top of the cake and dot whole almonds around the outer edge, if you wish. For an extra flourish, finely chop or ground another handful of almonds, mix with a pinch of cinnamon and sea salt and scatter all over the top.

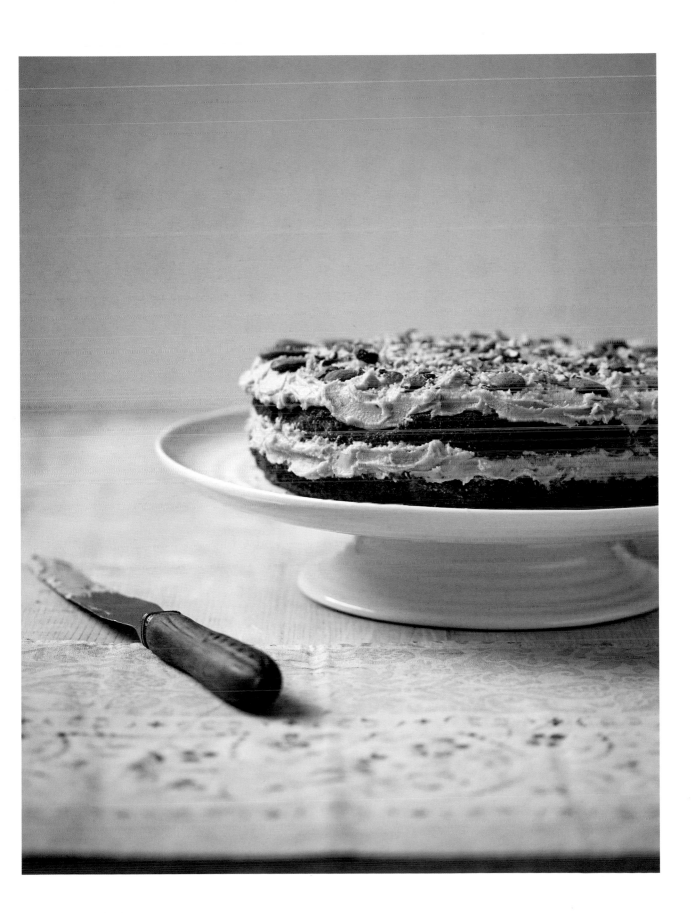

CHOCOLATE GINGER PEAR CAKE

Gluten-free. A dream to look at, heavenly to eat.

 0.5 PORTION
PER SERVING

PREP 20 MINS
COOK 45 MINS
SERVES 10

5 small ripe pears

zest and juice of 1 lemon

50g dark chocolate or
    unsweetened cacao,
    roughly chopped

150ml olive or almond oil,
    plus a little extra for
    greasing

50g cocoa powder

a thumb-sized piece of
    ginger, peeled and
    finely diced

3 eggs

½ tsp bicarbonate of soda

150g ground almonds

a pinch of sea salt

1 tsp ground cinnamon, plus
    extra for dusting

150g caster sugar or coconut
    palm sugar

Preheat the oven to 160°C/Gas 3.

Lightly oil a 23cm round or square cake or tart tin. Line the base with baking parchment.

Peel and halve the pears and use a teaspoon or small knife to carve out the seeds. Cut off the knobbly base and stalk at the top and place in a bowl with the lemon zest and juice to keep them from browning.

Place the chocolate or cacao in a little bowl over a simmering pan of water (making sure the water doesn't touch the base of the bowl). Stir until fully melted then set aside.

In a bowl, weigh 2 of the pear halves. You want 125g worth. If they're too big, cut a bit off until you get 125g worth. If they're not big enough, trickle in some of the lemon juice or a little water to bring the weight up to 125g.

Place your 125g of pears (and lemon juice/water, if used) with the oil, cocoa powder, melted chocolate and ginger in a blender or food processor and whizz until thick and creamy like chocolate mousse. Add the eggs and whizz again until everything is glossy, smooth and thick. Scrape the moussey mix into a large bowl.

Stir the bicarbonate of soda into the chocolate mix, then fold the ground almonds, salt, cinnamon and sugar through. Mix through until fully incorporated. Scrape the mix into your prepared tin.

Arrange the remaining 8 pear halves on top, cut side down. If using a round tin, have the narrow tops of the pears pointing toward the centre. The batter will rise up and edge them apart a little, so don't worry if they're a little close. If there's not enough room for all of them, just use what fits. If using a square tin, alternate them head to tail.

Place the tin on the middle shelf of the oven. Bake for 45 minutes, or until puffed up, toasty and set. Test the thickest part of the cake with the tip of a knife or a skewer – if it comes out clean, it's ready; if not, bake for longer and cover the top with foil if it's getting too bronzed.

Finish with a dusting of cinnamon, if you like. Delicious warm or cold.

MAMA MOORE'S APPLE CAKE WITH CARDAMOM AND WHITE CHOCOLATE

My colleague, Nicky Browning, at Abel & Cole introduced me to this marvellous cake when she brought it into the office to celebrate someone's birthday. As soon as I tasted it, I asked Nicky for the recipe, and I wasn't the only one. It's really unusual in that it starts out looking like pastry, and every time I make it my mind boggles at the vast quantity of apples packed into it and how, in the oven, it magically transforms into a cake. Mama Moore's original recipe didn't include the cardamom and white chocolate, and you can leave them out, or swap the cardamom for a different spice (fresh ginger, nutmeg, vanilla, fennel seeds, caraway). Mama Moore, by the way, is Nicky's mum.

 PORTION PER SERVING

PREP	30 MINS
COOK	40 MINS
SERVES	9–12

225g self-raising flour (or 220g plain white flour plus 1 tsp baking powder)

¼ tsp bicarbonate of soda

a pinch of sea salt

6 cardamom pods, seeds finely ground

100g cold butter, cut into small cubes

450g cooking or dessert apples

a little lemon juice

75g white chocolate, finely chopped (optional)

100g caster sugar or coconut palm sugar, plus extra for the top

2 eggs, beaten

Preheat the oven to 200°C/Gas 6. Lightly oil a round or square 23cm cake tin with a removable base.

Sift the flour, bicarbonate of soda, salt and cardamom into a mixing bowl and mix thoroughly. Add the butter cubes to the flour and rub into a breadcrumb consistency.

Peel and core the apples and cut into very small, thin pieces. Toss them in a little lemon juice as you go, to keep them from browning.

Fold the apples, white chocolate, if using, and sugar into the butter and flour mix. Gently fold in the beaten eggs until everything is thoroughly combined – do not beat the mixture; folding is the key to success.

Turn into the lightly oiled cake tin and level off the top of the batter. Sprinkle a little sugar over the top.

Bake for 30–40 minutes, or until golden on top and set in the centre. Insert the tip of a knife or skewer in the centre – if it comes out clean, it's ready; if not, bake for longer and cover the top with a piece of foil if it's getting too bronzed.

Remove from the oven and leave to cool before turning out onto a serving plate. Serve hot on its own or with a dollop of crème fraîche, yoghurt or mascarpone.

PUMPKIN IN A CHEESECAKE

Considering it has a whole pumpkin in it, this ghoulish creation errs on the healthier side of the spectrum.

 PORTIONS PER SERVING

PREP   30 MINS (PLUS CHILLING)
COOK   30 MINS
SERVES 8

1kg pumpkin or squash

a gloss of olive oil

200g walnuts, toasted

100g dates, pitted

1 tbsp cocoa powder

2 tsp ground cinnamon

75g soft brown sugar

1 tbsp vanilla extract, or
    seeds scraped from
    1 vanilla pod

1 tsp ground ginger

1 tsp ground nutmeg

1 tsp ground cloves

250g cream cheese, or make
    labneh with 500g natural
    yoghurt (see page 58)

250–300ml double cream

sea salt

Preheat the oven to 220°C/Gas 7. Put a large roasting tin in the oven to heat.

Cut the pumpkin or squash into wedges. Scoop out the seeds (save and toast for a snack) and gloss the wedges with oil. Add a pinch of salt and tumble onto the roasting tin. Roast for 30 minutes until mashably tender.

Whizz the toasted walnuts, pitted dates, cocoa powder, 1 teaspoon of the ground cinnamon and a little salt in a blender or food processor until fully ground. Press into a 20cm springform tin (or use 8–10 ramekins for individual cheesecakes) and chill.

Once the pumpkin/squash is cooked, scoop the flesh from the skin and whizz to a purée in a blender or food processor or using a hand blender. Add the sugar and remaining spices. One the mix is cool, whip in the cream cheese or labneh and cream. Taste, and add more spices, if needed. Once the mixture is thick, smooth and tasty, spread it over the chilled base.

Leave to chill for 4 hours in the fridge or for 1 hour in the freezer before serving.

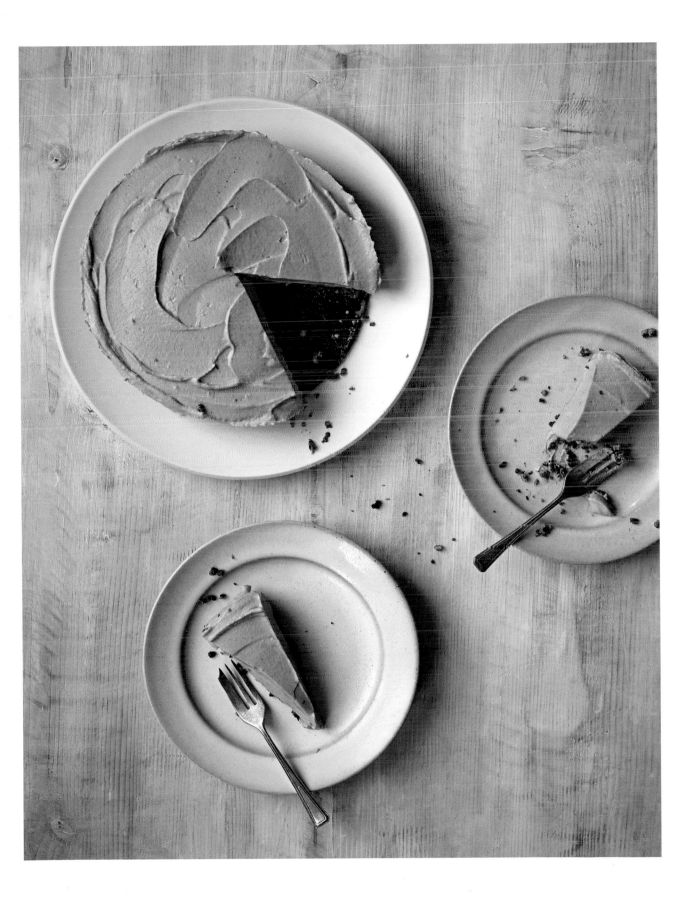

CARROT CAKE SCONES

Sugar-free, sprinkled with wholegrains, packed with a portion of fruit and veg and beautiful to eat – these scones have a lot going for them. Perfect for breakfast or as an afternoon treat.

 1 PORTION
PER SCONE

PREP   10 MINS
COOK   15 MINS
MAKES   6 MEDIUM-SIZED SCONES

100g plain white flour, plus extra for dusting

100g wholewheat or spelt flour

3 tsp baking powder

¼ tsp sea salt

2 tsp mixed spice

zest and juice of 2 oranges

3 tbsp raisins

50g cold butter, cut into small cubes

1 tbsp runny honey, plus extra to serve

1 large or 2 small carrots, coarsely grated

1 egg, to gloss the tops (optional)

mascarpone, to serve

Preheat the oven to 200°C/Gas 6. Grease and dust a baking sheet with flour.

In a bowl, mix the flours, baking powder, salt, mixed spice and the zest of one of the oranges.

In another bowl, add the raisins and the orange juice and set aside.

Toss the cold butter cubes through the flour. Work the butter through the flour using your fingertips (as if making pastry).

Drain the raisins, saving the juice. Swirl the honey into the juice and set aside. Fold the drained raisins and the carrots through the flour mix. Add 1 tablespoon of the honeyed orange juice at a time, until the flour forms a ball that's a little sticky but not too wet. You'll need about 5–6 tablespoons of juice to achieve this consistency.

Tip the dough onto a well-floured surface. Shape into a 3cm-thick rectangle and use a round cutter or the rim of a glass to cut out your scones. You should get about 6. Place on the prepared baking sheet, brush the tops with whisked egg for a glossy finish, and bake for 15 minutes in the centre of the oven, until golden and cooked through. Leave to cool for 5 minutes.

Fold the reserved orange zest into a little mascarpone and ripple through a drizzle of honey. Halve the scones and slather with the cream.

NOTE: I find scones are best eaten on the day they're made so I've gone for a small batch, but the recipe doubles easily. And if you make more than you need, just freeze the cooked or uncooked scones for another day.

Jelly

THE BASICS: Jelly is not just for children's birthday parties. It's refreshing, light and, using the following recipes as a guide, it can be rather healthy. Once you get the hang of making your own jelly, you can transform fresh juices or puréed fruits into healthy, wobbly puds that you can inject with spices, flowers and booze. I find the best setting agent is agar agar, which is derived from seaweed. It's easier and faster to use than gelatine, plus it's vegan and vegetarian friendly. It doesn't dissolve as beautifully, but I get around this by straining the liquid to remove any lumpy bits.

If your jelly doesn't set, simply reheat the mix with a little more agar agar. Strain, chill again, and hopefully that'll do the trick. If it has set too thick, simply reheat with some extra juice or whatever you used as your base and chill until it's ready to wobble.

ROSY POMEGRANATE PANNA COTTA

 PORTION
PER SERVING

PREP	15 MINS (PLUS 1 HOUR TO SET)
COOK	5 MINS
SERVES	4

500ml pomegranate juice

1 tbsp dried rose petals or rose water

seeds from ½ a vanilla pod or 1 tsp vanilla extract (optional)

2 tbsp agar agar flakes

2–3 tbsp runny honey, agave, sugar or your favourite sweetener

250ml crème fraîche, Greek or natural yoghurt

Warm the pomegranate juice with the rose petals or water, vanilla, agar agar and 2 tablespoons of the honey/sweetener. Whisk until the agar agar flakes have dissolved. Strain through a fine mesh sieve, scraping as much through as possible.

Whisk in the crème fraîche/yoghurt. Taste. Add a little more honey/ sweetener, if needed.

Divide between ramekins. I love using little jam jars or pretty tea cups.

Chill for 1 hour or until set. Scatter fresh pomegranate seeds or rose petals over to the top to garnish.

PLUM AND LIQUORICE

This jelly is full of fun, and fruit. The liquorice is a brilliant complement to the plums – sweet and aniseedy. A match made in heaven.

 PORTIONS PER SERVING

PREP 10 MINS (PLUS 1 HOUR TO SET)

COOK 5 MINS

SERVES 4

4 ripe plums, halved and stones removed

500ml apple juice (freshly squeezed, if possible)

2 liquorice sticks (the real thing, not the sweet), or 75g natural liquorice (the sweet), plus extra to serve

2 tbsp agar agar flakes

2–4 tbsp runny honey (if using the sticks)

Place the halved plums in a blender or food processor with the juice and whizz until smooth.

Pour into a saucepan with the liquorice sticks (or if using natural liquorice sweets, thinly slice them first before adding 50g) and agar agar and warm over a medium heat until the agar agar dissolves. Whisk vigorously a few times to help mix everything together.

Press through a sieve to strain out any lumpy bits of agar (scrape the bottom of the sieve to reclaim as much as you can) and whisk again.

Taste, and stir through enough honey or sweetener to suit (if using liquorice sweets, add more of these, if needed). Reheat gently, if needed, to help the agar dissolve further. Pour into glasses and pop into the fridge for about 1 hour to set. Top with some small chunks of natural licorice to serve.

PINEAPPLE AND STAR ANISE

This one packs a serious punch; star anise and pineapple were made for each other. If you've got a juicer, time and energy, definitely go for fresh juice. It's healthier by far and has a phenomenal flavour.

1 PORTION PER SERVING

PREP 5 MINS (PLUS 1 HOUR TO SET)

COOK 5 MINS

SERVES 4

750ml pineapple juice

4 whole star anise

2 tbsp agar agar flakes

1–2 tbsp runny honey or your favourite sweetener

Place the pineapple juice, star anise and agar agar in a saucepan. Warm over a medium heat, whisking until the agar agar has dissolved.

Press through a sieve to strain out any lumpy bits of agar (scrape the bottom of the sieve to reclaim as much as you can) and whisk again.

Taste, and stir through enough honey or sweetener to suit. Reheat gently, if needed, to help the agar dissolve further. Pour into glasses and garnish with a star anise in each glass, if you like. Pop into the fridge for about 1 hour to set.

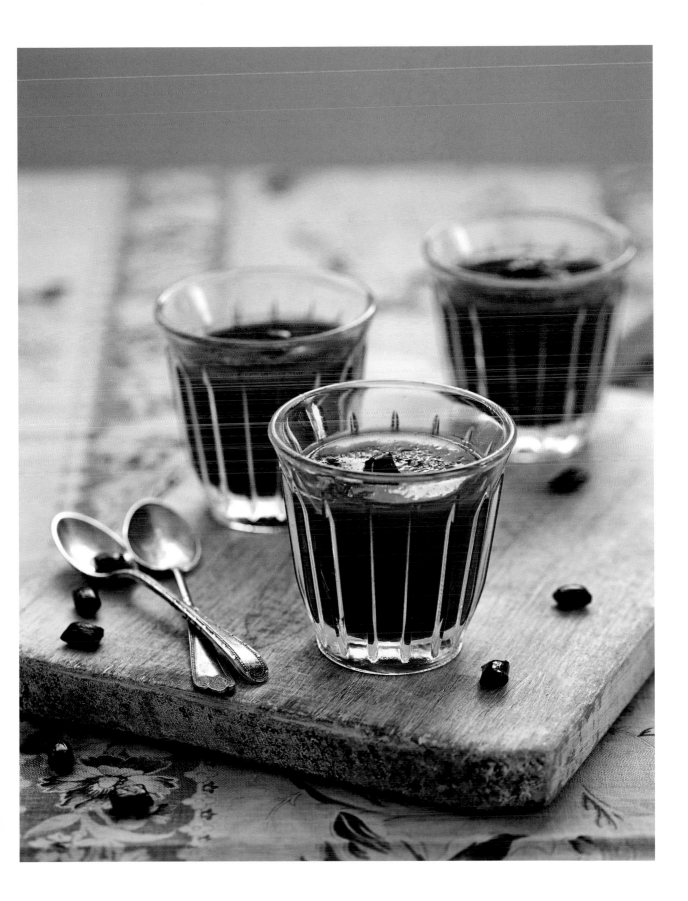

APPLE ELDERFLOWER JELLY

This is just one twist on an apple-juice-based jelly. There are endless options: swapping the elderflower for blackcurrant cordial, mango juice for lime and fresh mint, or adding spices, herbs or other fruits.

 PORTION PER SERVING

PREP 5 MINS (PLUS 1 HOUR TO SET)

COOK 5 MINS

SERVES 4

750ml apple juice

50ml elderflower cordial (more or less, to taste)

2 tbsp agar agar flakes

a few fresh elderflowers, to garnish (optional)

Place the apple juice in a saucepan with the elderflower cordial (tasting as you trickle the elderflower in until the sweetness and flavour is just right – the strength varies according to make). Once it's just right, add the agar agar and warm over a medium heat, whisking until the agar agar dissolves.

Press through a sieve to strain out any lumpy bits of agar (scrape the bottom of the sieve to reclaim as much as you can) and whisk again.

Reheat gently, if needed, to help the agar dissolve further. Pour into glasses and pop into the fridge for about 1 hour to set. Garnish with fresh elderflowers, if you can get some.

JAFFA JELLY

This jelly was inspired by the mighty Jaffa Cake. If you've got any leftover vanilla or plain sponge cake, set a thin sliver in the bottom of each glass before pouring the chocolate over, although the creamy chocolate ganache alone is delicious and evocative enough of the classic biscuit to satisfy.

 PORTION PER SERVING

PREP 15 MINS (PLUS 1 HOUR TO SET)

COOK 5 MINS

SERVES 4

75g dark chocolate, finely chopped

a good pinch of ground cinnamon

35ml freshly boiled water, cooled very slightly

750ml orange juice (freshly squeezed, if possible)

1 fresh bay leaf (optional)

2 tbsp agar agar flakes

2 tbsp runny honey

Place the chocolate in a heatproof bowl with the cinnamon. Swirl the boiling water into the chocolate, stirring until the chocolate is fully melted, thick and glossy. Spoon the chocolate into the bottom of 4 glasses and place in the freezer to set.

Place the orange juice in a saucepan with the bay leaf (tear it around the edges a couple of times to release its flavour) and the agar agar and warm over a medium heat, whisking until the agar has dissolved.

Press through a sieve to strain out any lumpy bits of agar (scrape the bottom of the sieve to reclaim as much as you can) and whisk again.

Taste, and stir through enough honey or sweetener to suit. Reheat gently, if needed, to help the agar dissolve further. Leave the jelly to cool a little, and your chocolate to set further, before pouring the orange jelly on top of the chocolate. Pop into the fridge for about 1 hour to set.

Poached

THE BASICS: Poaching fruit is gorgeous. It's like enrobing it in flavoured silk. Use beautifully ripe, seasonal fruit, with its own built-in sweetness, and you only need the tiniest drop of honey or sugar. You also won't need to poach the fruit for too long, just simmer until the flavour of your poaching liquid has married with your fruit. You can use any liquid to poach your fruit – beer, tea, wine, fruit juice, cordial or even water – and you can add spices and sweets (I'm thinking liquorice), herbs and flowers (lavender or rose petals).

OH MY DARLIN' CLEMENTINES

This is a recipe with two tales: a tipsy Spanish one, and a healthy South African one. The first traces back to my love of Spanish food: pairing citrus with a sweet sherry and Marcona almonds just makes sense. The second was born when I brewed up a pot of rooibos tea far greater than I could sip. I tossed in a cinnamon stick and a few orange slices and created a delicious marriage of flavours.

 PORTION PER SERVING

PREP   5 MINS
COOK   15 MINS
SERVES 4

8 small clementines or 4 oranges, peeled and cut into 2cm-thick slices

750ml strongly brewed rooibos tea or 250ml sweet sherry, such as Oloroso

1 stick of cinnamon

a drizzle of runny honey or your favourite sweetener (optional)

a handful of salted or roasted Marcona almonds, roughly chopped or crushed (optional)

Place the clementine or orange slices in a saucepan. Cover with the tea or sherry and add the cinnamon stick. Gently simmer over a low heat for 15 minutes, or until the oranges have lapped up the flavour of the tea or sherry.

Taste, and swirl in a little honey or sweetener, to suit. Leave the flavours to infuse a little if you're not serving straight away. Can be served hot or cold with a dusting of almonds over the top, if you like.

HONEY BLOSSOM PEACHES

This stunning little dessert is so simple, elegant and beautiful. It relies on ripe and sweet peaches, so if your fruit is not quite there on the sweetness front, roast them in a 180°C/Gas 4 oven until soft, sticky and sweet. Then poach them in the honeyed blossom water below, just long enough to tickle them with its flavour.

1 PORTION PER SERVING

PREP 15 MINS
COOK 10 MINS
SERVES 4

600ml water

2 tbsp runny honey (more or less, to taste)

1 tbsp orange blossom water

4 ripe peaches

Place the water, honey and orange blossom water in a saucepan large enough to hold the peaches. Bring to a simmer over a medium heat, whisking to dissolve the honey.

Add the peaches. Simmer for 10 minutes, or until softened. Remove from the heat and leave to steep for a further 10 minutes.

Spoon the peaches out of the pan and slip them out of their skins, squeezing any excess juice from the skins before discarding. Place each peach in a bowl. Spoon some of the poaching liquid over and serve.

MULLED FIGS WITH MASCARPONE

1 PORTION PER SERVING

PREP 10 MINS
COOK 25 MINS
SERVES 4

350ml red wine●

1 tbsp runny honey or brown sugar

½ a vanilla pod, split open and seeds scraped out

2 star anise

1 cinnamon stick

3 black peppercorns

6 cloves

2 bay leaves

12 fresh figs

mascarpone, to serve (optional)

Place the wine, honey, vanilla, spices and bay leaves in a saucepan. Warm over a medium–low heat. Halve the figs vertically, slicing through the stalks so they're identical on both sides. Lower them into the mulling wine. Gently simmer for 20 minutes, or until the wine is infused with the spices and the figs are tender and saturated with the spiced wine.

Divide the figs and their poaching liquid between bowls or wine glasses and serve with a dollop of mascarpone, if you wish.

● *For an alcohol-free alternative, swap the wine for pomegranate juice.*

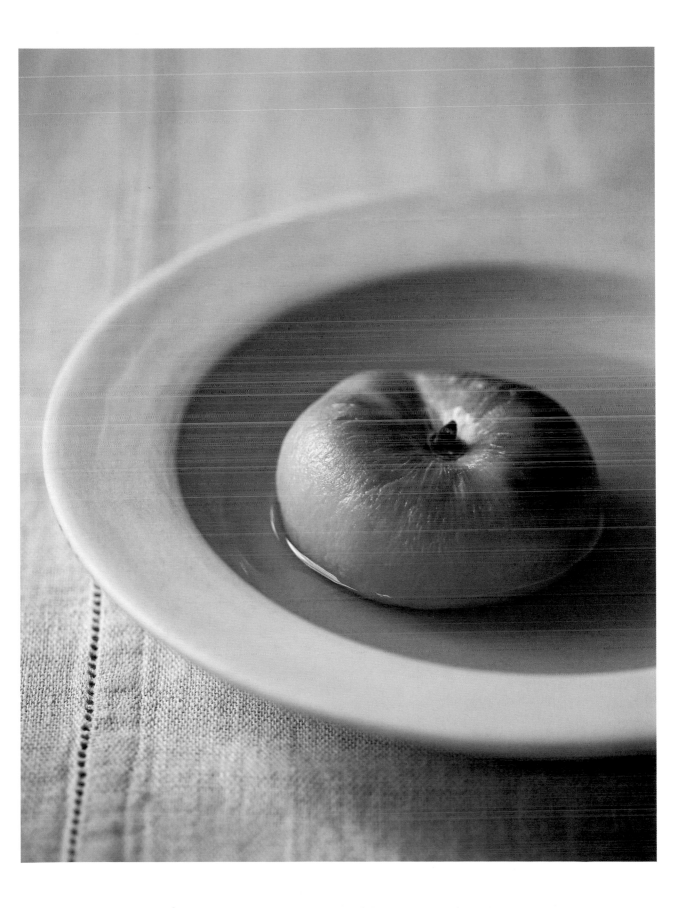

CHOCOLATEY PEARS

While whole poached pears look pretty, you need a heap of poaching liquid to cover them, they take an age to poach to perfection and you don't get as rich a flavour as you do when you poach slices of pear instead. Try it – it'll become a favourite. The cocoa recipe here is based on an eighteenth-century recipe I learned at the historic Hampton Court Palace.

 1 PORTION PER SERVING

PREP 15 MINS
COOK 15 MINS
SERVES 4

6 tbsp cocoa powder

1 tsp vanilla extract, or the seeds scraped from ½ a vanilla pod

½ tsp ground cinnamon

a pinch of chilli powder

a pinch of ground Szechuan pepper (optional)

500ml boiling water

a splash of milk or cream

2 tbsp runny honey or your favourite sweetener (more or less, to taste)

4 ripe pears (ideally Conference pears)

Put the cocoa, vanilla, cinnamon, chilli and Szechuan, if using, into a saucepan. Slowly whisk in the water until dark, thick and a little frothy. Sweeten to taste. Trickle in a little milk or cream to round the flavour and soften the richness.

Peel the pears and cut into 3cm-thick slices, carving out the core when you get to it. Gently lower the slices into the simmering hot chocolate. Simmer until the pear slices are soft and infused with flavour, about 10 minutes. Taste one of the slices to make sure it's just right.

Spoon the chocolatey pear slices into bowls or pretty cups. Pour some of the warm chocolate sauce over. Beautiful on its own, or serve with vanilla ice cream, mascarpone or crème fraîche.

GINGER BEER POACHED RHUBARB

 1 PORTION PER SERVING

PREP 5 MINS
COOK 15 MINS
SERVES 4

320ml ginger beer

1 tbsp runny honey

400g rhubarb, cut on the diagonal into 3cm hunks

Pour the ginger beer and honey into a saucepan. Simmer over a medium heat until the honey has dissolved, stirring often.

Lower the rhubarb into the warm liquid. Poach until the rhubarb is just tender, about 10 minutes.

Spoon the rhubarb into dishes with some of the poaching liquid. Gorgeous with a dollop of clotted or thick whipped cream, or a scoop of vanilla ice cream.

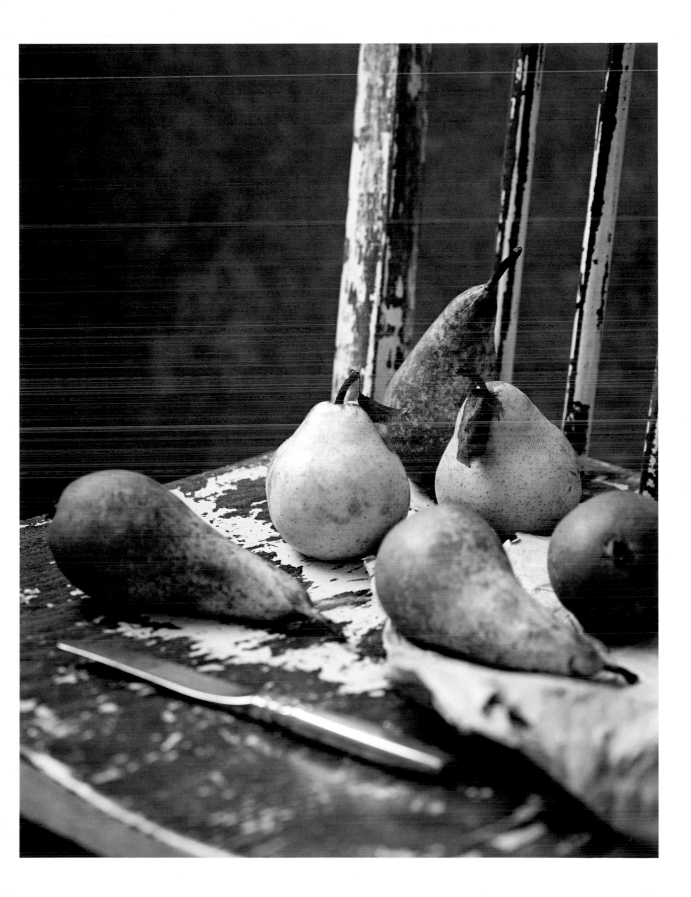

Chocolate Fondue

THE BASICS: This is a brilliant way to get fruit into little tums. It's equally popular with adults, and is great fun to dish out at the end of a meal if you've got friends over – or even just to brighten a work night.

You really can't go wrong with silky melted chocolate. Even if you're on a strict sugar-free diet, you can indulge by sourcing pure cacao over chocolate and letting the fruit do all the sweetening.

The fondues here are basically melted water-ganache truffles with hint of spice, nuts or other fragrant things. Water and chocolate mix as beautifully as cream and chocolate – almost better, in fact. If your mix splits (probably due to your water being too hot), just grab a whisk and whip it firmly until everything mingles back together.

SEPI'S SALTED CURRANTS WITH ROSE CHOCOLATE POTS

Every time I see my Iranian friend Sepideh Black, she inspires me with either an amazing recipe idea or a genius gardening trick. One of the many wonderful things Sepi has taught me is that redcurrants are amazing with a little pinch of sea salt. That little pinch of salt makes the fruits burst to life. In keeping with the flavours of Sepi's motherland, I've paired her beautiful currants with a rose-infused dark chocolate fondue.

1 PORTION PER PERSON

PREP	10 MINS
COOK	5 NIL
SERVES	4

100g dark chocolate

⅛ tsp rose water

50ml hot water

350g redcurrants

a pinch of sea salt

Roughly chop or break the chocolate up and place in a heatproof bowl. Add the rose water, swirl in the hot water and stir until all the chocolate has melted and the mix is creamy and silky smooth. Set the bowl over a simmering pan of water, if necessary, to help it melt further.

Place your mini chocolate fondue in a pot in the centre of the table or in individual espresso or similar-sized cups.

Rinse the redcurrants. Sprinkle with a little sea salt and serve alongside the fondue for dipping.

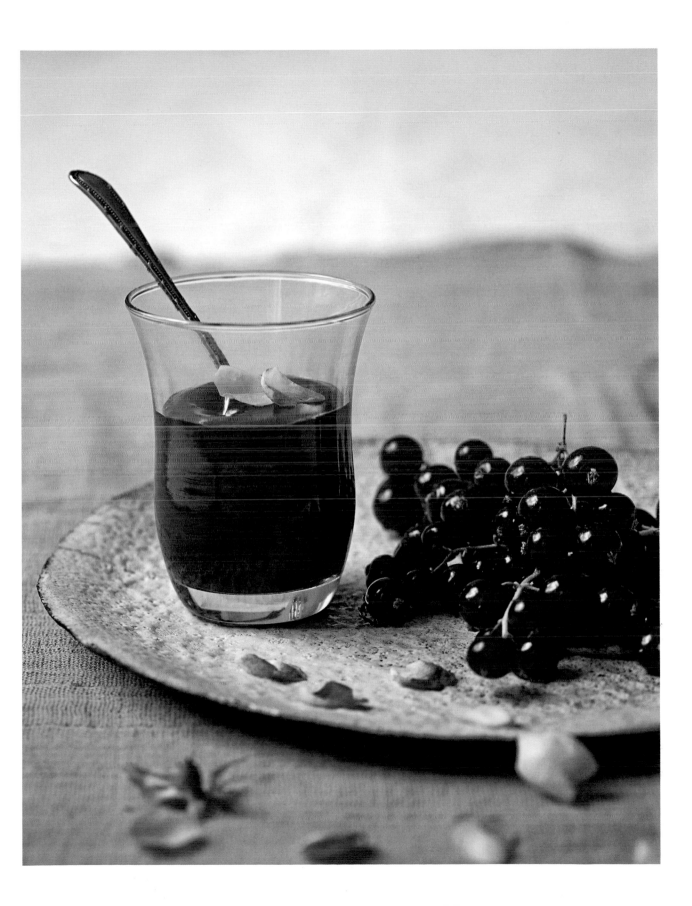

BLACK PEPPER CHOCOLATE WITH STRAWBERRIES

This recipe started as a fresh mint chocolate fondue with strawberries, but the mint just wasn't coming through. So I started thinking of all the other things strawberries love. Balsamic works well with strawberries, but my word it does not go with chocolate. A good pinch of black pepper, however, set the world right again. Strawberries, black pepper and chocolate: a trio to make your heart sing.

PORTION PER PERSON

PREP   10 MINS
COOK   NIL
SERVES 4

100g dark chocolate

a good pinch of black
   pepper (to taste)

a pinch of sea salt

50ml hot water

350g strawberries (trimmed
   and skewered or just
   served whole)

Roughly chop or break the chocolate up and place in a heatproof bowl. Add a pinch of pepper and salt, swirl in the hot water and stir until all the chocolate has melted and the mix is creamy and silky smooth. Set the bowl over a simmering pan of water, if necessary, to help it melt further. Taste, and add a little more pepper, if needed.

Place your mini chocolate fondue in a pot in the centre of the table or in individual espresso or similar-sized cups.

Serve with the whole or trimmed and skewered strawberries.

MELTED PEANUT BUTTER CUP WITH FROZEN BANANA LOLLIES

My son's not wild about bananas, so we tend to end up with a fruit bowl full of soft, speckled fruit. I use them to make instant banana lollies to dip into this moreish fondue. Now this he does go bananas for.

PORTION PER PERSON

PREP   20 MINS (PLUS
        FREEZING TIME)
COOK   NIL
SERVES 4

4 bananas, cut into 3cm
   chunks

100g milk chocolate

25ml hot water

1 tbsp peanut butter

a pinch of ground cinnamon

Wiggle the hunks of banana onto skewers, 2–3 hunks on each skewer, giving each person 3–4 skewers each. Freeze on a greaseproof paper-lined baking tray for 1–2 hours.

Roughly chop or break the chocolate up and place in a heatproof bowl. Swirl in the hot water and stir until all the chocolate has melted and the mix is creamy and silky smooth. Set the bowl over a simmering pan of water, if necessary, to help it melt further. Swirl the peanut butter and cinnamon into the melted chocolate.

Place your mini chocolate fondue in a pot in the centre of the table or in individual espresso or similar-sized cups. Serve with the frozen banana lollies for dipping.

CHERRIES WITH MOCHA

Coffee and cherries is a magical mix. In fact, coffee beans actually grow inside a cherry-like fruit. In its dried form, it's called cascara and can be brewed into an amazing tea. It has a really delicate cherry-like flavour, disguising the fact that it has way more caffeine than coffee. If you can get some, and if you can handle a caffeine roller coaster, swap the coffee in this recipe for cascara. If you're a caffeine wimp like me, however, go for a coffee substitute like chicory, dandelion or simply opt for decaf.

 PORTION PER PERSON

PREP 10 MINS
COOK NIL
SERVES 4

100g dark chocolate

seeds from ½ a vanilla pod, or 1 tsp vanilla extract (optional)

50ml hot, freshly brewed coffee

350g cherries (pitted and skewered or just served whole)

Roughly chop or break the chocolate up and place in a heatproof bowl. Add the vanilla, if using, swirl in the hot coffee and stir until all the chocolate has melted and the mix is creamy and silky smooth. Set the bowl over a simmering pan of water, if necessary, to help it melt further.

Place your mini chocolate fondue in a pot in the centre of the table or in individual espresso or similar-sized cups.

Serve with the whole or stoned and skewered cherries for dipping.

CARDAMOM WHITE CHOCOLATE WITH FIGS

This is a classic, first introduced to me by the wonderful Chantal Coady, founder of Rococo Chocolate. Chantal has been a wonderful friend in the world of chocolate over the years. She taught me how to temper chocolate, has lent me cacao pods from the Grenada cacao farm she works with and, most importantly, has inspired me with all sorts of wonderful flavours.

 PORTION PER PERSON

PREP 10 MINS
COOK NIL
SERVES 4

100g white chocolate

3 cardamom pods, seeds finely ground

a pinch of sea salt

25ml hot water

350g ripe figs (trimmed and skewered)

Roughly chop or break the chocolate up and place in a heatproof bowl. Add the cardamom and a pinch of sea salt, swirl in the hot water and stir until all the chocolate has melted and the mix is creamy and silky smooth. Set the bowl over a simmering pan of water, if necessary, to help it melt further.

Place your mini chocolate fondue in a pot in the centre of the table or in individual espresso or similar-sized cups.

Serve with the whole or trimmed and skewered figs for dipping.

Frozen

THE BASICS: I've gone for simplicity and minimalism here. A beautiful sweet treat need not be laden with sugar or require lots of fussing over, especially when you're using beautiful sun-kissed seasonal fruit. There's something quite magical about a frozen dessert. The following fruits are completely transformed once frosty.

FROZEN BLACKBERRIES WITH HAZELNUT CHOCOLATE SHARDS

I discovered this dessert by accident. I had a punnet of blackberries from my local allotment squirrelled away in my freezer, tumbled them into a bowl to thaw out, but my son and his friend almost finished the lot immediately. They were like self-contained sorbets, frosty but still full of the sweetness from the late summer sun.

 PORTION PER SERVING

PREP   10 MINS (PLUS OVERNIGHT FREEZING)

COOK   5 MINS

SERVES   4

350g blackberries

100g dark chocolate

50g hazelnuts, roughly crushed or chopped, toasted

Rinse the berries and pop them in the freezer for at least 2 hours, or ideally overnight.

Set a glass or metal bowl over a saucepan of gently simmering water. Add two-thirds of the chocolate to the bowl and stir until it has fully melted. Take the chocolate off the heat and swirl in the remaining chopped chocolate until it melts into the mix.

Place a sheet of greaseproof paper on a baking tray. Pour the chocolate onto it, scatter the toasted nuts on top and pop into the fridge or freezer to set.

Once it's ready, break into shards and serve alongside the chilly berries (take them out of the freezer and pop them in a bowl 10 minutes before serving).

PEACH JULEP

I make this one without the bourbon twist for my son. Indeed, you can go for complete purity by simply grating a frozen peach or nectarine. I just pop the entire fruit, skin and all, into the freezer, and before grating I run the fruit under warm water and the skin slips off with a little help from your fingers.

 PORTION PER SERVING

PREP   10 MINS (PLUS FREEZING TIME)
COOK   NIL
SERVES 4

4–6 ripe peaches (or nectarines)

4 fresh mint leaves

a drop of bourbon (optional)

1 tsp brown sugar (optional)

Freeze the peaches or nectarines until solid.

Stack the mint leaves on top of one another. Roll them up like a cigar and thinly slice.

Run the fruit under warm water for a second, then slip the skins off and coarsely grate.

Divide the fruit between dishes. If you're going for the julep twist, add a few drops of bourbon (½–1 tsp per serving) over the icy fruit. Dust with brown sugar and finish with wisps of mint.

LASSI LOLLY

My son eats curry at a push, but the promise of one of these at the end of a meal is the bait I use to lure him. It reels him in every single time – the perfect refreshing finish to a spicy Indian meal.

 PORTION FOR LARGER LOLLIES/0.5 PORTION FOR SMALL LOLLIES

PREP   15 MINS (PLUS FREEZING TIME)
COOK   NIL
SERVES 4–8 (DEPENDING ON THE SIZE OF YOUR LOLLY MOULDS)

300g ripe mango, peeled and cubed●

2 cardamom pods, seeds finely ground

200ml natural or Greek yoghurt

1 tbsp runny honey or your favourite sweetener

Place everything into a blender or food processor and whizz until smooth. Pour into your ice lolly moulds and freeze until fully set.

> ● *This recipe relies on a buttery, sweet mango. If you cut into it and it's a bit tangy or tough, I'd give it a miss and use 300g peeled bananas instead.*

ASIAN MELON ICE POPS

You can turn just about any juice or smoothie into an ice lolly. This is one of my favourites – and a great way to get kids to eat melon.

 PORTION PER ICE POP

PREP 15 MINS (PLUS FREEZING TIME)
COOK NIL
SERVES 4

½ ripe Galia, Charentais, Cantaloupe or Honeydew melon, seeds discarded

1 tsp runny honey or your favourite sweetener (more or less, to taste)

½ tsp freshly grated ginger

a squeeze of lime juice

Scoop out the flesh of the melon and pop it into a blender or food processor. Add the honey or your chosen sweetener, ginger and a squeeze of lime juice, and whizz to a purée.

Taste, adjust the sweetness to your liking, and pour into ice lolly moulds. Freeze for at least 3 hours or until frozen solid. When ready to eat, run under a little warm water to help loosen from the lolly mould.

APPLE SNOW

This is my version of granita. Rather than making a flavoured sugar syrup and breaking it up with a fork, I tried grating frozen fruit to achieve the same effect. It worked and tastes heavenly. The texture is soft like snow. It tickles your tastebuds and then, like magic, disappears in your mouth.

 PORTION PER SERVING

PREP 15 MINS (PLUS FREEZING TIME)
COOK NIL
SERVES 4

4 apples

Pop the apples in the freezer until solid, peel (from frozen), then coarsely grate. Or freeze large peeled hunks of apple and grate them in your food processor if you have a grating attachment. Work quickly and serve them up as each apple is grated or they'll thaw before you're done.

NOTE: I've tried these little mounds of apple snow with a drop of rose water and various spices, but the apple sings on its own.

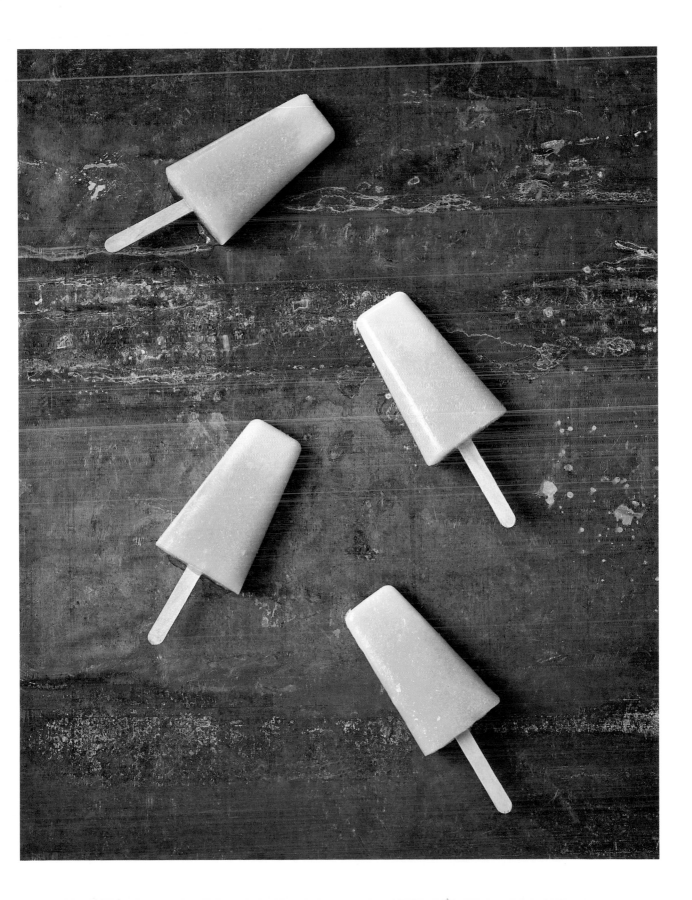

INDEX

ACKNOWLEDGEMENTS

My gorgeous son Rory has two cracking recipes in this book – his Gingerbread Ice Crème and his Jerk Lamb are both corkers. He's been an enormous part of this book's evolution, trying every single recipe in the book at least once, as well as sampling the flops that didn't make it. He's also been incredibly patient as I disappear into the kitchen for hours; taking far too long to get his dinner on the table and making him late for school due to recipe testing his breakfast.

Much love and thanks go to my husband for all of his support and to my mother who has nurtured my lifelong love of fruit and veg. As well as my mother, my granny and granddad, Ima and Lloyd, and my siblings Robin, Marshall and Skipper who forever inspire and feed me with their phenomenal cooking.

Huge thanks to my Crystal Palace friends, especially to my dear friends Karen Jones & Laura Marchant-Short who run the amazing Crystal Palace Food Market, which supplied much of the food for the recipe testing and photoshoots. Special mentions to Clare, Robin and Rochelle at Patchwork Farm, Paul and Jason at Brockman Farm, Wade Taylor from the Grain Grocer, Jayne & Michael Duveen from Jacob's Ladder Farms, Adrian Izzard of Wild Country Organics.

Enormous thanks to ALL OF MY lovely colleagues at Abel & Cole, especially Yuriko Matsukawa and Lauren Hyde, who came along to the shoots to help with food styling and the washing up! Yuriko's amazing work can be seen on the cover! Also to Philip Cowell, Nicky Browning (and her mum, Mrs Moore), Gary Congress, Paul Freestone and Jassy Davis for recipes and endless inspiration.

When it comes to getting your little ones to eat more fruit and veg, Lucy Thomas is the expert. My section on Children & Veg was initially four-pages long and much of it included invaluable tips from Lucy. Do get her book *Mange Tout: Teaching Your Children to Love Fruit and Vegetables Without Tears* (Penguin; 2007). It's a life changer.

Last but certainly not least, I am forever grateful to the enormously talented Sarah Lavelle who fought to make this book happen, and to the team who made it all come to life: the wonderful Nassima Rothacker and her assistant Simon Mackenzie for all the luscious photographs, David Eldridge and his team at Two Associates, and Charlotte Portman, Louise McKeever and the rest of the team at Ebury. Thank you!